RISK MANAGEMENT IN HEALTHCARE ORGANIZATIONS

CARMEN RAIMONDO

I dedicate this work to my wonderful family

Strengthening the principles of ethics and moral integrity,
by health and management professionals,
is necessary to put the health, safety and welfare of patients above all else and to improve the quality of care at all levels.

INDEX

LIST OF TABLE   **10**

LIST OF FIGURE   **12**

INTRODUCTION   **13**

CHAPTER 1   CORPORATE RISK

1.1 Definition   17
1.2 Types of risk   20
References   24

**CHAPTER 2   THE PROCESS AND ELEMENTS
              OF RISK MANAGEMENT**

2.1 Risk management as a continuous process   25
2.2 The phases of Risk Management Process   30
    2.2.1 Enterprise Risk Management model (ERM)   30
    2.2.2 Sustainable Enterprise Risk Management
       (SERM)   41
2.3 Benefits and limits   44
References   46

CHAPTER 3 RISKS AND ERRORS IN HEALTHCARE

3.1 Risk management in healthcare organizations   47
3.2 Risk Mapping: identification of critical areas   54
3.3 The problem of errors in the exercise of healthcare
    activity   59
    3.3.1 A classification   59
    3.3.2 Risks of particolar gravity: Sentinel Events   65
References   70

CHAPTER 4 STRATEGIC PROCESS OF RISK MANAGEMENT

4.1 Strategic Process   73
    4.1.1 Why Risk Management in Health Care?   73
    4.1.2 Risk Management steps: using the ERM model
    in the Health Care System   80
4.2 Prevention strategies and risk reduction   96
    4.2.1 Guidelines and Recommendations   98
References   103

CHAPTER 5 OPERATIONAL INSTRUMENTS FOR RISK MANAGEMENT

5.1 Risk identification tools   105
    5.1.1 Incident Reporting   105
    5.1.2 Reporting by Users   111
    5.1.3 Civic Audit   113
5.2 Towards a reactive and proactive risk analysis   115
    5.2.1 Root Cause Analysis   115
    5.2.2 FMEA (Failure Mode and Effect Analysis)
    and FMECA (Failure Mode, Effects and
    Criticality Analysis)   120
5.3 Risk treatment tools   124
    5.3.1 The use of innovative computerized
    technologies to improve security and safety   124
    5.3.2 Case Study: San Raffaele Hospital, Milan   126
References   129

**CHAPTER 6   RISK MANAGEMENT IN
INTERNATIONAL AND
NATIONAL   CONTEXT**

6.1 The US context from the '70s to today   131
6.2 The situation in Italy   136
    6.2.1 National initiatives about Risk Management   136
    6.2.2 New rules on Risk Management and
        responsibility of health professionals
        (Law March 8, 2017, No 24)   140
    6.2.3 A survey on health care organizations   142
        6.2.3.1 Risk Management in the Italian
            healthcare context   142
        6.2.3.2 Areas, tools and techniques of Risk
            Management   153
References   156

CONCLUSION   157

LIST OF TABLES

Table 1.1   ERM- Enterprise Risk Management Model   19
Table 1.2   Speculative or strategic risks   22
Table 1.3   Pure risks or threats   23

Table 2.1   Objectives   27
Table 2.2   Strengths and weaknesses   28
Table 2.3   External and internal factors   34
Table 2.4   Description of the risk   35
Table 2.5   Risk assessment   36

Table 3.1   Clinical risk factors   50
Table 3.2   Risk based on the type of accident   51
Table 3.3   Hygienic and environmental risks   52
Table 3.4   Risk factors   52
Table 3.5   Structural risks   53
Table 3.6   Organizational risks   54
Table 3.7   Analysis of the main claims for compensation for Specialties/ Services   56
Table 3.8   Areas of Risk and Claims for compensation   58
Table 3.9   Errors in medicine in the United States   60
Table 3.10 Theory of errors (Reason)   61
Table 3.11 Types of errors (general and specific errors)   62
Table 3.12 Claims Analysis by type of events and errors (Hospital)   64
Table 3.13 Type of Sentinel Event-2004/2014 (JCAHO)   67
Table 3.14 Type of Sentinel Event (2015, 2016, 2017)   68

Table 4.1   Elements of the ERM model   81
Table 4.2   Activities and functions of the URM   86
Table 4.3   Contributing factors   88
Table 4.4   Quantitative assessment   92
Table 4.5   Assessment matrix of quantitative risk   92
Table 4.6   Qualitative assessment - Estimation of damage severity   93
Table 4.7   Qualitative assessment-Estimated probability of occurrence (expressed as number of errors per 100 admissions)   94
Table 4.8   Characteristics of the Guidelines   100
Table 4.9   Examples of recommendations   102

Table 5.1   Strengths and Weaknesses   108

Table 5.2   Types of events (adverse events/near miss)   109

Table 5.3   Reporting Hospitals /Local Health   113

Table 5.4   Example of FMEA / FMECA application in Anesthesia   122

Table 6.1   Recommendations 2005-2014   137

Table 6.2   Risk Management in Italian healthcare Organizations   144

Table 6.3   Areas deemed to be at risk for the company X   153

Table 6.4   Areas of implementation of Risk Management projects   154

Table 6.5   Adoption of tools for reporting errors   154

Table 6.6   Risk Management Techniques   155

LIST OF FIGURES

Figure 2.1   Pre-analysis of the business organization   29
Figure 2.2   SERM Model   43

Figure 3.1   Claims for compensation   58

Figure 4.1   Quality is improved by integrating the
             different dimensions of a system   76
Figure 4.2   The safety culture and context factors behind
             an effective risk management process   79
Figure 4.3   The process of Health Risk Management   82
Figure 4.4   Structure of Corporate Risk Management   84
Figure 4.5   Structure of the Risk Management Unit   84
Figure 4.6   Structure of Committee For Claims
             Assessment   85
Figure 4.7   Sources for risk identification   87
Figure 4.8   Example of analysis of adverse event   91

Figure 5.1   Types of User Reports and Reports used by
             Public Relations Offices   112
Figure 5.2   Reason's Model   116
Figure 5.3   Root Cause Analysis process (RCA)   117
Figure 5.4   Diagram of Ishikawa   119
Figure 5.5   FMEA/FMECA Process   121
Figure 5.6   Drug Mistakes   126

Figure 6.1   The management methods used   143
Figure 6.2   The total/partial adoption of Risk
             Management model   149
Figure 6.3   The timing of implementation of Risk
             Management projects   150
Figure 6.4 a Obstacles to implementation by type of
             Projects (Risk Management and Total
             Quality Management)   150
Figure 6.4 b Obstacles to implementation by type of
             Projects (Balanced Scorecard and Lean
             Thinking)   151
Figure 6.5   Staff engagement strategies   152

INTRODUCTION

The topic of risk management in healthcare is closely related with the need to manage safety within the entire healthcare organization, both during the time spent in the structures that in the care delivery process. In fact, the risk is inherent in every level of the organization and it results from a number of factors, internal and external to the company.

Increasingly, reference is made to the concept of risk to a "global" level, to underline the fact that management have the task of examining all the events from which, actually or potentially, may arise a number of risks that hinder the achievement of set goals and which may put into question the overall strategy pursued by the company, which protects both individual and community.

In this context, the challenge for management is to identify a comprehensive and integrated approach able to:
- determine and manage risks arising from: a) socio-economic system in which the company operates (*external risks*) and b) organizational risks, which potentially contribute to erode the value created by their strategic and operational decisions (*internal risks*);
- provide adequate responses to reduce, remove and sometimes even to share the negative impacts resulting from the occurrence of unwanted and adverse events.
The latter do not facilitate the creation and maximization of value but affect the existing one.

For this reason, the problem of risk has become extremely important in healthcare nationally and internationally, for which the primary objective is the spread of so-called *"safety culture"* that produces implications for both staff and patients.

For staff of all levels and responsibilities, this means, on the one hand, to reinforce the principles of ethics and integrity, to place patient health and safety as the central factors in the process; the other, in creating a suitable working environment to carry out often complex tasks, that are not supported by a structure consistent with really performed activities. Consider, for example, the lack of communication between different specialties or even among health professionals of the same department.

For the patient it means treatment efficacy, improved quality of life in the long term, safety in the place where the patient is cared for and assisted.

This work aims to analyze the main strategies and techniques of treatment, reduction and elimination of health risks which, frequently, resulting mistakes and often irreparable damage but predictable, to prevent the likelihood or recurrence of the problem and consequences.

The first and second chapter focus attention on the concept of corporate risk in general terms, about the characteristics of the risk management system and elements that help to set it up.

In the third chapter we analyze how to manage risk in the healthcare system; it will attempt to identify the most critical areas and risks related to them.

The fourth chapter introduces the topic of risk management as a strategic process and it provides a description of prevention strategies and risk reduction more commonly used.

The fifth chapter analyzes the steps of risk analysis and identification of risk, risk treatment actions to be undertaken and the tools to be adopted to reduce, correct and gradually eliminate errors emerged in business and clinical processes.

Finally in the sixth chapter we proceed to a brief analysis of the risk management process in the US context. The same attention is focused on the evolution of this process in Italian Local Health, by presenting the results of an empirical study carried out between 2011 and 2014, to verify the development level of risk management process implementation.

CHAPTER 1

CORPORATE RISK

Summary: 1.1 Definition - 1.2 Types of Risk - References

1.1 Definition

In general, from a semantic point of view, the risk can be defined as the likelihood that a damage, an accident, an injury will occur, with an impact such as to prevent or adversely affect the achievement of the objectives.

Within the company it expresses the probability that a damaging event will occur, contrary to the expectations and strategies pursued. It may be the result of an individual action or, as is often the case, it may be due to system dysfunction.

In particular, it is frequently due to a defect in the organizational structure and infrastructure, or operational process of planning and control. In any type of business, the risks are both internal and external to the system and can contribute to modifying expected outcome of the system itself.

From a practical point of view, total risk elimination is not always a feasible solution, as it depends on the complexity of the system, in which each company operates, on the management decisions (*strategic risk*) and dynamism of the economic, social, political and technological context that may (positively or negatively) affect strategy implementation (*pure risk*)[1].

Enterprises that implement *Enterprise Risk Management* model (whose goal is to support value and competitive advantage created by them, par. 2.2.1) tend to classify all the internal and external events, resulting in potential development opportunities, but also risks that affect the growth, profitability, value creation, continuous improvement and innovation in management methods (tab. 1.1)[2].

Corporate level risks derive from the interaction between management decisions and actions and changes in the external environment.

Tab. 1.1 *ERM- Enterprise Risk Management Model*

CATEGORIES OF EVENTS	
External factors	**Internal factors**
Economic	**Infrastructure**
- Availability of capital	- Availability of material
- Issuance of loans, insolvencies	resources
- Concentration	- Potential of material
- Liquid assets	resources
- Financial markets	- Access to capital
- Unemployment	- Complexity
- Competition	
- Mergers and acquisitions	**Personnel**
Environmental	- Potential for human resources
- Pollution and waste	- Fraud
- Energy	- Health & Safety
- Natural Catastrophes	
- Sustainable Development	**Process**
Geopolitical	- Resources
- Changes in the political context	- Drawing
- Legislation and public policies	- Performing
- Regulation	- Providers
Socio-cultural	
- Demographic	**Technology**
- Customer behaviours	- Data integrity
- Company Nationality	- Availability of data and
- Privacy	systems
- Terrorism	- System selection
Technological	- Development
- Interruptions	- Diffusion
- E-commerce	- Maintenance
- External data	
- Emerging technology	

Source: PricewaterhouseCoopers, Il Sole 24 Ore, 2006[2]

Risk is perceived as a potential damage to the company. It must be distinguished from the concept of *"acceptable risk"*. According to a common definition given by the Committee of Sponsoring Organizations of the Treadway Commission (CoSO), *acceptable risk* is the amount of risk that a company is willing to accept in order to pursuit the value creation; it is consciously assumed by the management in response to environmental uncertainty, to produce differential values.

This implies that no one is able to completely remove any risk factor, as it is an integral and inevitable part of any context. It is intended to move forward with the rapid increase in complexity of the structures and increasingly advanced technology and instruments.

The aim is to develop a safety-oriented strategy, consistent with an acceptable level of risk, allowing the company to achieve its goals and mission, to evaluate the threats of a complex system composed of multiple components and to define the essential tools for achieving risk reduction to desired levels.

1.2 Types of risk

Any business context is not just a production function, but it is the result of strategic choices and changes in the external environment, depending also on the different risk profiles of the company's system.

Because of the greater environmental complexity (such as the processes of market integration and globalization and technological innovation), new types of risk have emerged in recent years. These have led companies to change their risk management strategy, to deal with such uncertainties and their effects.

It follows a concept of enterprise capable of foreseeing and counteracting a set of heterogeneous risks connected to each other, each of which is capable of transforming itself into an extraordinary event that could undermine the company's performance and success.

The different types of risk exposure are to be attributed to a single risk that is defined *"global risk"*. There is a close mutual dependence between them but also an overlapping of these types.

Although the analysis of the various risk concepts is usually carried out in a separate way, it is important to keep in mind that in the business practice an integrated risk management approach is adopted: this is to emphasize the company's ability to cope with all possible negative impacts, coming from inside or outside to it.

It is crucial to identify risks and threats that can damage the heritage of resources and skills, decrease the value and hinder the ordinary course of business. This allows to have a clear vision and knowledge of the risks throughout the organization.

It is possible to distinguish the following risk classes:

1) speculative or strategic risks;
2) pure risks or threats.

Speculative or strategic risks are closely related to strategic business management. They are divided into three categories (strategic, operational and financial ones) and they accompany almost all management decisions (risks related to advanced technologies, R&D activities and production processes, market risks, interest rate variation)[3]. They can result in both losses/threats and profit opportunities (tab. 1.2).

Tab. 1.2 Speculative or Strategic Risks

FINANCIAL RISKS	PRODUCTION RISK
- Economic Liquidity and Investments - Loan cost - Insolvency debtors - Change in interest rates	- Availability tangible and intangible resources - Appropriate technologies - Malfunctions/warehouse Failures
MARKET RISKS	TECHNOLOGICAL RISKS
- Change in market share - Change user preferences - Financial markets turbulence - Labor market turbulence and supplies - Exchange rate change - Interest rate change - Price change	- Unexpected technological Changes
SECTOR RISKS	STRUCTURAL RISKS
- Technological changes - Investments in R & D	- Incorrect sizing of technical, administrative and service structures
POLITICAL AND SOCIAL RISKS - Political instability - Failure to comply with the law - Corruption - Social instability - Lack of values and moral integrity	RELATIONAL RISKS - Unsatisfactory business climate - Reduced customer satisfaction - Lack of communication
REGULATORY RISK	RISKS OF IMAGE
- Tax, Legal, Regulatory	- Reputation and Reliability
COUNTRY RISK	ORGANIZATIONAL RISKS
- Currency risk - Commercial risk - Tax risk	- Strenuous Work Processes - Complexity of tasks - Lack of planning and control - Lack of training and Education

Source: adaptation by Zattoni, 2006, Il Sole 24 Ore

Pure risks always have a negative impact on both corporate assets (theft, fire) and integrity and health of third-parties (occupational illness and accidents) and in no case do they create a profit for those who endure it. These threats may have an intentional or accidental origin and they are characterized by the unpredictability that makes management difficult (tab. 1.3).

Tab. 1.3 Pure Risks or Threats

PROPERTY RISKS	SAFETY RISKS AT WORK
- Fire - Theft - Industrial espionage - Cybercrime - Sabotage	- Accidents - Professional illness
RISKS OF CIVIL LIABILITY TO THIRD PARTIES - Charges for contractual liability	ENVIRONMENTAL RISKS - Violation of environmental legislation - Natural catastrophes - Ecological accidents
RISKS OF INTERRUPTION OF ACTIVITIES - Blackout	

Source: adaptation by Zattoni, 2006, Il Sole 24 Ore

Both types of risks expose companies to uncertainties about achieving their planned strategic and operational goals. They involve a reduction in corporate assets and represent the so-called *"risk profile"* for the many risks associated with adverse events; these are due to mistakes made by individual operators and organizational system and they are determined by the external environment or by technology[4].

References

1. ZATTONI A., (2006), *Corporate Governance,* Collana Management, Il Sole 24 Ore.
2. PRICE WATERHOUSE COOPERS, (2006), *La Gestione del Rischio Aziendale ERM. Enterprise Risk Management: modello di riferimento e alcune tecniche interpretative,* Il Sole 24 Ore.
3. FLOREANI A., (2004), *La valutazione dei rischi e le decisioni di risk management,* EDUCatt Università Cattolica.
4. MESSINA G., (2014), *Economia e organizzazione delle aziende sanitarie,* Libreria Universitaria Ed. Webster Srl, Padova.

CHAPTER 2

THE PROCESS AND ELEMENTS OF RISK MANAGEMENT

Summary: 2.1 Risk management as a continuous process - 2.2 The phases of the Risk Management process. *2.2.1 Enterprise Risk Management model (ERM) 2.2.2 Sustainable Enterprise Risk Management (SERM)* - 2.3 Benefits and limits - References

2.1 Risk management as a continuous process

Enterprises operating in a competitive and dynamic environment must face uncertainty about achieving its strategic and operational goals. Effective strategic management is the means by which management is able to anticipate the response to changes in the context in which it operates, in order to address the long-term goals it intends to achieve.

It is a continuous process of adaptation since, in the event of unforeseen changes, the enterprise must review:

- the plans related to its strengths and weaknesses;
- its ability to compete;
- opportunities and external threats;
- actions to be taken in the expected times.

So, once the strategy is selected, it is necessary almost always to change it. In fact, new opportunities and threats make it ineffective for the purposes for which it was designed and planned. This principle is also valid for internal management system, oriented to the effective

performance of business functions and their integration[1].
Risk management system is placed in this context.

Risk Management is a continuous and systematic
process through which management seeks:

- to actively address uncertainties and related risks and
  opportunities that are reflected in many ways on the
  priority objectives;
- to design control systems for coping with risk
  situations, minimizing the possibility of errors and
  maximizing the ability to generate value and
  preserve it over time.

Integrated risk management system is a widely
recognized model since it examines the risks and
opportunities that affect value creation and value
maintenance.

It can be defined as follows: "it is a continuous
process, put in place by Board of Administration,
management and other professionals in an organization,
to formulate strategies designed to identify potential
events that may affect the business, to manage risk
within the limits of acceptable risk and to provide
reasonable assurance that the entity's objectives will be
achieved"[2].

From this definition we can see that the borderline
between business strategy and risk has become more and
more limited and it is crucial to consider and analyze
both aspects in an integrated way, to get an advantage in
achieving the predefined business goals (tab. 2.1).

Tab. 2.1 Objectives

Strategic	High-level objectives to support the company mission
Operational	Effective and efficient management of business resources, including mechanisms of protection from losses
Reporting	Reliability of internal and external information (accounting and non-accounting)
Compliance objectives	Compliance with reference standards (civil, fiscal, ethical, labor, environmental)
Objectives of business protection or resource protection	They are aimed at preventing losses of assets due to theft, waste and any inefficiency generated by imprudent management

Source: PricewaterhouseCoopers, Il Sole 24 Ore, 2006

In addition to being aimed at achieving these goals, an effective risk management process creates a competitive advantage, increases stakeholder value, allows successful exit from adverse situations and often difficult to foresee.

Continuous business strategy development and review is carried out simultaneously with the analysis and management of potential risks, through a continuous series of actions that interact with each other, involving all the activities carried out at strategic and operational levels.

The risk management model is a continuous, constant and pervasive process; for this reason it encourages staff at every level, within the organization, to gain a

27

proactive and shared risk insight.

In this regard, it may be useful to identify possible strengths and weaknesses in the Risk Management process (tab. 2.2).

Tab. 2.2 Strengths and Weaknesses

STRENGTHS	WEAKNESSES
It analyzes the problems from different points of view	Inability of the company to deal with unidentified or minimized threats
It identifies the activities that limit the risk, formulating appropriate responses	Improper allocation of resources with disproportionate costs for marginal risk
It seizes potential opportunities without limiting risk identification	
It improves the quality of decision-making processes	

Integrated risk management is a natural evolution in management practices. In fact, by identifying, analyzing, evaluating and eliminating these risks, they are aimed at defining corrective actions and improving business processes, so that the organization can minimize losses and maximize opportunities (fig. 2.1).

Fig. 2.1 Pre-analysis of the business organization

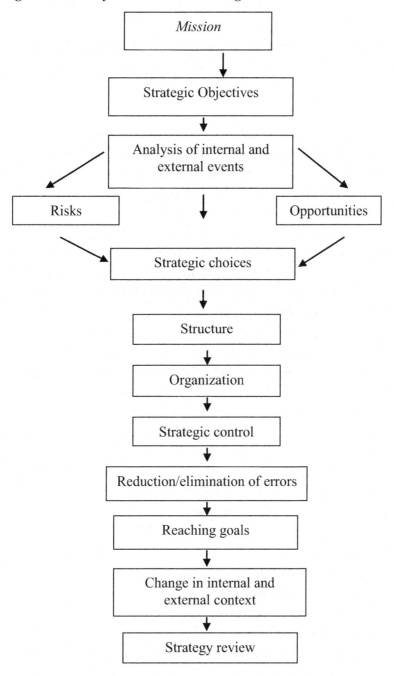

2.2 The phases of the Risk Management process

2.2.1 Enterprise Risk Management model (ERM)[2]

The corporate risk management model is the result of a project started and backed up in 2001 by the Committee of Sponsoring Organizations of the Treadway Commission (CoSO). The objective was to achieve a significant benchmark for all business entities, regardless of their sector of affiliation, size, culture and management philosophy, including all types of risk, their identification and management processes.

This document is defined as ERM (Enterprise Risk Management). It represents a review of the previous one *"Internal Control System"* and it strengthens the issue of risk assessment as a crucial prerequisite for an effective control system planning. It can be adopted both as an internal control tool and to acquire a full knowledge of the risk management process.

This model supports the management in taking decisions that are considered more appropriate to minimize the effects of adverse events and to determine, as a final result, a reasonable assurance of achieving planned strategic goals.

Regardless of the type of company in which it is implemented, it is the combination (not necessarily sequential) of eight elements:
1) internal environment;
2) goal setting;
3) identification of events/risks;
4) risk assessment;
5) risk response actions;
6) control activities;
7) information and communication;
8) monitoring.

Each of these elements interacts with others and it is incorporated in the context of actions and decisions taken by management. This model pursues the goal of developing capabilities:

- for knowing the enterprise in its entirety, in terms of mission, strategies, goals, organizational structure, operating mechanisms;
- to integrate risk management in daily operational and management practices, since risk and control are activities that involve and concern everyone.

In this perspective, the model provides tools to identify and deal with unexpected external and internal events, enhancing the ability to know in advance the impact of a future event. The essential features of the elements mentioned above will be described below.

1) Internal environment

Internal environment is the main element of the risk management model, as it concerns the attitude of the organization in the face of the probability that one or more events may compromise the implementation of business strategies. Therefore, the elements that contribute to its configuration are not just the people working within the structure but, in particular, the way in which they act and assume the resulting responsibilities of their actions.

The staff will share not only the same values and behaviors, on how to achieve the goals, but also a management philosophy designed to better identify, understand, evaluate and govern the different risk profiles, both at a single operating unit level and at company level. This is desirable insofar as:
a) the company can rely on a quality management system, characterized by ethical behaviors, managerial and entrepreneurial skills;

b) it is possible to have a good organizational structure that defines authority positions, roles, responsibilities, solid trust relationships and effective communication systems;

c) resource training policies are geared towards enhancing the knowledge and skills of staff so that they can adapt effectively to change and address risk factors, many of which are unstable and increasingly heterogeneous.

This model must be supported by a culture of integrity and ethical values, for which staff are required to act legally and morally, promptly reporting serious adverse events and risk situations before they pose a significant threat to the organization.

2) Goal Setting

The goals, which are relevant for risk management, include strategic and related ones.

Strategic goals are general ones and they are consistent with the corporate mission, with which the company aims to achieve competitive advantages and create value.

Related goals support the strategic ones and they are determined later. They concern:

a) effectiveness, efficiency of business operations and how the resources are allocated (*operational goals*);

b) the effectiveness of the information system, created by internal and external data (*reporting goals*);

c) compliance of business activities with laws and regulations (*compliance goals*).

It is essential to define these goals clearly for an effective identification of all events, which may result in risks and threats of varying magnitudes. They must therefore be formulated in a clear, realistic and correct way, in order to ensure optimal allocation of resources between different operating units. To each objective is assigned a percentage of risk set by the company (*acceptable risk*) that it is willing to bear for carrying out its mission and take new initiatives.

It is obvious that the company will take on greater risk by pursuing an innovation strategy aimed at continuous improvement and by developing, for example, new services rather than maintaining the quality of existing ones.

In this context, the risk management system does not provide guidance on what objectives to achieve, but it ensure an alignment of the objectives with the company's mission and consistency with the acceptable risk level decided by the company.

3) Identification of events

This phase requires an in-depth analysis of all internal and external factors that can generate critical events and thus an accurate knowledge and analysis of the organization and its external environment (tab. 2.3). It is also important to look at events that could have a significant impact on planned targets, although they are less likely to occur.

It is necessary to distinguish between the analysis of the current environment (and its impact on current strategies) and the analysis of the future environment in which the company will face unforeseen and unforeseeable situations.

Tab. 2.3 External and internal factors

EXTERNAL FACTORS	INTERNAL FACTORS
Economic	Infrastructures
Environmental	Personnel
Political	Process
Social	Technology
Technological	

In this process, the company adopts techniques that allow to identify both past events (through historical data collection), which have generated losses and future events that have not been previously experienced, through the acquisition of information from external sources, considering the likelihood of occurrence and impact.

The most frequently used methodology is the "*mapping risks*" or "*claim register*". It provides information about:

a) the most frequent areas of risk, the types of events that have occurred or are unusual and related consequences (damage to persons and property);

b) the possible action priorities for improving processes and staff safety.

Subsequently, a detailed description of each identified risk factor can be made, through tables that are useful to place it in a specific category (tab. 2.4).

Tab. 2.4 Description of the risk

NAME OF RISK	- - - - -
PURPOSE OF RISK	Qualitative/quantitative description of events, number and type
NATURE OF RISK	Strategic, operational, financial, knowledge, compliance
STAKEHOLDER	Stakeholder and their expectations
RISK QUANTIFICATION	Relevance and probability
RISK TOLERANCE	Potential and financial risk impact. Identification of the desired level of performance
CONTROL MECHANISMS AND RISK TREATMENT	Identification of protocols for review and monitoring
POTENTIAL ACTIONS OF IMPROVEMENT	Recommendations to reduce the risk
DEVELOPMENT STRATEGIES AND POLICIES	Identification of function responsible for developing strategies and policies

Source: IRM , AIRMIC; 2002, *A risk management standard*[3]

4) Risk Assessment

Risk assessment is a continuous process of action on business activity, aimed at verifying the positive or negative impact of a potential event on achieving the goals. It is implemented through the identification of sources of danger; it is based on the collection of information about internal and external situations (work, change in environmental legislation, etc.) that may create risks in the activity carried out. The following examples relate to the assessment of organizational risks and risks of workers' health (tab. 2.5).

Tab. 2.5 Risk assessment

Source of risk	Characteristics	Assessment
Security procedures	Disposal of hazardous waste	Are there corporate procedures?
Exposure to biological agents	Transport of material (blood)	Is there a suitable container that complies with regulations for transport in the laboratory?

Source: Risk Assessment Document, Local Health Reggio Emilia[4]

For an effective assessment, potential risks are grouped in categories of homogeneous event (organizational, economic, worker health, safety) and are examined both at the level of a single operating unit and at company level. Risk assessment and measurement (strategic, economic or operational ones) can be achieved quantitatively and qualitatively.

The most used quantitative techniques are benchmarking, probabilistic and non-probabilistic models.

In literature, *benchmarking* has been defined as a systematic and continuous process of information gathering and analysis, aimed at comparison between different organizational units of a company or between a company and other similar ones that represent the "excellence [..] in achieving the best performances"[5].

The objective is to identify appropriate performance measures, which can be expressed through a complete system of indicators[6].

Indicators express the strategic, organizational and economic performance of the company as a whole and its operating units. Examples of indicators are:
a) percentage incidence of staff on revenues;
b) percentage incidence of material on revenues;
c) percentage incidence of maintenance on revenues;
d) average cost of staff;
e) number of administrative positions compared to the total staff.

The comparison with indicators system and performance standard of other similar companies allows to identify any critical areas to be subjected to further verification, in order to take actions for improving management and organizational processes.

Probabilistic models evaluate the risk based on:
a) chance of occurrence of an event: remote, occasional, probable, frequent;
b) consequential impact: no damage, slight damage, no serious damage. They use simulations of expected results and future trends (level and quality of services and benefits provided, research and development costs, staff training).

An appropriate criterion should be defined beforehand to make a representation of the envisaged scenarios, ensuring maximum transparency of the assumptions made.

Finally, non-probabilistic or subjective models are used only to estimate the impact of a potential event but not the probability of occurrence.

Qualitative techniques are used to analyze the factors that could represent a business risk (image problems, regulatory requirements, etc.). They are based on subjective judgments by evaluators, who must have an extensive knowledge of the potentially adverse events. Generally, they involve risks:

a) which cannot be estimated with a reasonable approximation;
b) whose consequences cannot be measured reliably;
c) which require a very burdensome search and analysis of reliable data.

5) Risk response actions

After identifying and assessing risks, containment actions must be defined, depending on the company's risk appetite. The basic principles of risk management forecast to face the risk, according to a defined logic sequence:

a) *Elimination*: the aim is to anticipate through planning the occurrence of uncertainty or triggering events, thus canceling the effect as well. For example, the company might decide not to engage in new initiatives that are considered highly risky or to replace a process that is too dangerous.
b) *Reduction*: if the solution given in the above first step is not reasonably possible, safety measures should be foreseen to deal with residual dangers, in line with the risk tolerance. In this case, it might be useful to balance the resources between the different operating units, assign greater responsibility to the management in decision making processes and in monitoring phase and enhance security systems.
c) *Transfer*: if there is a residual risk, part of it must be shared by subscribing an insurance policy for unexpected damages; contractual agreements with other companies; outsourcing of operational processes.

d) *Tolerance*: in this case, the company takes on its own risk (in part or in total), self-insuring against losses.

Based on the information acquired, it is possible to take the most appropriate and economically advantageous alternative, assessing the costs that must be sustained in terms of staff, processes, technology and compare them to the benefits that come with it.

6) Control activities

After the phase of risk treatment, all the steps described above should be reviewed over time to ensure that the solutions adopted are effective, efficient and realistic with respect to business objectives and, if necessary, take corrective action.

Controls can be preventive, concomitant and subsequent and they are implemented throughout the whole organization. They may concern:

a) the cost-effectiveness of management operations, in terms of effectively achieving the expected economic outcomes and rational use of available resources;
b) the reliability of business information system and the communication process of the information produced;
c) compliance with applicable laws, both legislative (fiscal, civil, environmental, work safety) and voluntary systems (quality certification, ethical standards).

7) Information and communications

At this stage, the most important information, about internal and external management, needs to be identified, recorded and communicated in the ways and times required, to make the staff aware and responsible for their tasks. They relate not only to economic and financial information, but also information to routine activities, staff management, applicable law, draft laws and user preferences.

The complex system of information often can be traced back to an advanced technology infrastructure (Information Technology) that allows to find, process, analyze real-time data, spread them in the right times, make them available at any point in the organization and to the right people. This contributes to reducing the uncertainty associated with development of increasingly complex relationships and operations.

Clearly, it is important to acquire and disseminate relevant and quality information for management and staff, as it enables the control of the whole business process management and all risk profiles associated with it.

However, having information is not sufficient for managing uncertainty. In fact, they have to go across the whole company, both vertically and horizontal (continuous communication between the different hierarchical functional areas).

In particular, a regular and continuous communication, (through meetings and discussions between management and staff), can facilitate the strengthening of the risk management system and corporate culture values, as well as the identification of new events.

8) Monitoring

The entire risk management process must be continuously monitored in order to make corrections if necessary. Monitoring activity is integrated into business management system and can be carried out with continuous or separate evaluations. Continuous assessment concerns the observation of activities carried out during the current management within the different operating units and it is rooted in business processes (acquisition of new customers, analysis of the economic and financial situation, check of the correct application of rules and regulations, updating and training courses).

It focuses attention on dysfunctions found at the different levels and allows to find out how the staff has acted against them and difficulties encountered during their control activities.

Separate assessment is a periodic activity in the event of changes in strategy, structure and system security; it consists of a series of actions that affect the entire company or specific management areas and all stages of risk management. Often it may be a self-assessment process in the context of their activity and their specific objectives.

Any shortcomings that have emerged must be referred through reports to all workers directly responsible for the process (direct superior, top management and board of directors). They will have issue directives, how to intervene and the consequent corrective actions to be taken.

2.2.2 Sustainable Enterprise Risk Management (SERM)[7]

Although little mentioned in the literature, it should be stressed how some companies have implemented a *sustainable* ERM model (SERM), that represents an extension of the traditional one. It is commonly referred to as a sustainable risk management system that includes categories of social and ethical risk and key areas, in a context where companies must operate in a wider competitive environment:
- external environment;
- organizational culture;

- staff recruitment based on merit criteria and protection of the human rights in the workplace;
- internal and external health and safety.

The goal is to achieve practical benefits in all key areas of reference, to create a sustainable organization capable of dealing with any type of adverse event and to provide other benefits (in addition to the concrete reduction of risks) such as:
- protection and improvement of the corporate image;
- recruitment and retention of talented staff;
- development of innovative services.

A SERM Sustainable Strategy is focused on the following aspects:
- the role of people in the business planning process, assessment, risk analysis and formulation of a risk strategy (*people and plans*);
- personal responsibility and communication of corporate risk profile at all levels;
- a careful analysis of all business processes and not only of those in which errors are more frequent;
- achieving performance in the areas considered, in a highly integrated way with the vision and business goals (Fig. 2.2).

Fig. 2.2 SERM Model

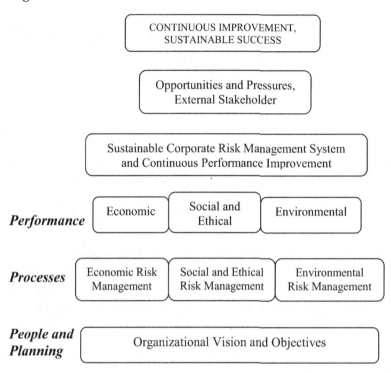

Source: adaptation by Spending e Rose, 2008

Within the model, the most important aspects are the social, cultural and ethical ones. The underlying idea is that these elements will help to reduce the distortions and adverse events present at every level of the structure, orienting the corporate strategy to a recovery of principles and values not only in individual subjects, but in the internal and external interaction of the organization.

2.3 Benefits and limits

Risk Management process is a strategic and transversal tool for corporate governance; it should be managed by top management, to identify all events that can cause damage and loss of any entity.

It is a new methodological approach, adopted as a response to changes produced by new business models and technologies; it allows to highlight the evolution of risk exposure over time, by indicating and quantifying improvements, compared to similar companies.

Regardless of the methodology used, the model allows to define what you want to protect from risk, identify and decide what threats to face, calculate residual risk in the limits of the risk considered acceptable by the company.

This should encourage process makers to create a common language of risk management, considering it not only as a tool to avoid making mistakes, but above all to guide people to make the right decisions, consistent with the obstacles that can be envisaged.

In fact some events are uncontrollable, but an accurate knowledge of the own organization and respect for shared rules, on the way of achieving general and specific goals, can help to improve response to the risk identified, reducing negative impact and consequential losses.

Applying this model will enable all stakeholders to gain a global view of the company and relationships with external stakeholders, through a more effective communication and addressing their action plans towards the goals set.

This does not mean that an effective Risk Management system is always fit for the purpose for which it has been prepared, as there is no certainty that uncontrollable or unpredictable events cannot occur (human error, error of judgment, malfunction of a technology, scarcity of resources, violation of policies and procedures established for illegal purposes, such as altering the economic and financial situation or non-compliance with legal provisions).

However, a well-designed risk management system can contribute, on the one hand, to reducing the occurrence of errors at individual, organizational (work context) and inter-organizational levels; on the other, to increasing protection of the system, optimizing interactions between all human activities, business culture, technology, organization and external environment.

Indeed, each person acts in relation to other individual and/or group, in turn, related to procedures, rules, technological processes, external subjects, environmental factors. When these elements and interactions between them are badly designed, failure of the whole system can emerge, which can be answered through the rule of learning by error.

Intervention actions focus not so much on who has caused the event, but on the underlying organizational and management factors related to communication, information exchange, training, roles and responsibilities.

These factors trigger dangerous situations throughout the organization, when associated with local factors (active mistakes of operators).

References

1. PELLICELLI G., (2006), *Strategia*, Collana Management, Il Sole 24 Ore.
2. PRICE WATERHOUSE COOPERS, (2006), *La Gestione del Rischio Aziendale ERM. Enterprise risk management: modello di riferimento e alcune tecniche interpretative*", Il Sole 24 Ore.
3. THE INSTITUTE OF RISK MANAGEMENT (IRM), The Association of Insurance and Risk Managers (AIRMIC), (2002), extract of the document *A Risk Management Standard*.
4. ASL REGGIO EMILIA, (2013), *Documento di Valutazione dei Rischi*, Aggiornamento 14.02.2013.
5. CASANOVA T., DE VITA A., (2007), *La gestione della conoscenza nelle PMI*, Franco Angeli Ed.
6. REGIONE EMILIA ROMAGNA, (2004) – Progetto di ricerca finalizzata, *Benchmarking su Indicatori di performance clinica, organizzativa ed economica delle Aziende Ospedaliere Universitarie Italiane*.
7. SPEDDING L., ROSE A., (2008), *Business Risk Management Handbook - A sustainable approach*, Elsevier Ltd.

CHAPTER 3

RISKS AND ERRORS IN HEALTHCARE

Summary: 3.1 Risk management in healthcare organizations. - 3.2 Risk Mapping: identification of critical areas. - 3.3 The problem of errors in the exercise of healthcare activity. *3.3.1 A classification. 3.3.2 Risks of particular gravity: Sentinel Events* - References

3.1 Risk management in healthcare organizations

The risk problem in healthcare has highlighted the need of modern health systems to govern the complexity of the many human, organizational and technological elements that characterize them; this urges them to achieve high standards of quality, in line with patients and healthcare professionals' expectations.

Risk is the main object of study of the healthcare system, both from an epidemiological point of view and in terms of action and prevention. In fact, in general the concept of risk is closely related to the health and safety of people and to all situations that may cause a decrease or loss.

Even in healthcare, it is defined as the likelihood of a danger to health and safety and not just as an obstacle to the achievement of goals that may hinder the delivery of effective care and services to people (the concept of *"global risk"*, which is borrowed from other organizational contexts).

For this reason, healthcare systems are increasingly pursuing and sustaining a stable policy of continuous improvement of safety within structures, identifying and controlling conditions and factors that can cause harm to the patient, to all those who work in them and to minimize the occurrence of errors and accidents.

Health risk analysis comprises the medical care dimension and organizational management one. The most common intervention areas of risks are: (Albergo F., 2014):[1]

1) **Clinical Risk and Pure Clinical Risk**: risks related to accidental damage; risks related to the user and then associated with delivery of healthcare services (surgical, diagnostic and therapeutic errors, infections);

2) **Chemical and biological Risk**: risks related to safety and protection of medical staff and patients;

3) **Organizational and Structural Risk**: risks related to the work environment, physical state (environmental risk) and structures management (technical risk and risk asset), plants and company assets.

Clinical risk lies in the broader and complex health care system and it has always been a delicate issue for both patients and all health care professionals.

The most commonly definition used is the following: "the risk is the likelihood that a patient is subjected to an adverse event, injury or discomfort, a deterioration of health or death, attributable to the medical care provided, even if involuntarily, during hospital stay period"[2].

A more specific and rigorous definition is provided by a document of the WHO, which states that "the risk is a probability of an undesirable event or a predictable or unforeseeable damage caused by healthcare management and related to every aspect of care delivered to a patient, from diagnosis to treatment, from systems and equipment used for care"[3].

From this it emerges that the context of healthcare is embodied in a series of activities and processes of care that can be traced back to a dense network of interactions between individuals, groups of individuals, rules, choices and managerial decisions that contribute to the delivery of care.

Consequently, the risks for patients are mainly due to procedural and organizational problems, to careless behaviors and to a legislation that discourages competent bodies from acting effectively. Factors that affect clinical practice and that are closely related to clinical risk are described below (tab. 3.1).

Tab. 3.1 Clinical risk factors

FACTORS	DESCRIPTION
Institutional context	- Economic context - Rules of the NHS
Management and organizational factors	- Resources and financial constraints - Policies, strategies and objectives - Culture of security and priorities
Work environment	- Staffing and skills - Workloads and shifts - Design and maintenance of equipment - Administrative and management support
Factors related to the work team	- Verbal and written communication - Supervision and seeking help - Team structure
Factors related to Individuality of the staff	- Knowledge and skills - Motivation - Ethics of behavior - Physical and mental health
Factors related to the task	- Design and structural clarity of the task - Availability and use of procedures - Availability and accuracy of test results
Patient characteristics	- Conditions of complexity and seriousness - Language and communication - Personality and social factors

Source: Vincent C., Adams S.T., Stanhope N., BMJ, 1998[4]

Chemical and biological risks are also defined as hygienic and environmental risks or health risks. They can be described as the likelihood of developing a disease, almost always infectious, due to exposure to chemical and biological agents and generated by equipment, plant, process and operating modes. They are responsible for any damage caused to personnel involved in hazardous operations, activities and process that exposes them to environmental, chemical and biological factors[5].

This type of risk also affects patients, because of the typical nature of diagnostic and care functions, characterized by a close relationship between them and the operators, each of which can become a potential source of risk for the other, even through the use and exposure to devices or equipment that often require an adequate staff training for their proper use.

Additionally, most infections are recorded in laboratory personnel, pathology anatomy, operating room and first aid (with serious consequences for patients in the last two cases).

The following are the results of a research on potentially transmissible risks, based on the type of injury (tab. 3.2), as well as a classification of more frequent risk factors that can be attributed to an unsuitable hygienic and environmental conditions (tab. 3.3).

Tab. 3.2 Risks based on the type of accident

Exposure mode	Risk of infection
Deep wound caused by a hollow needle	High
Contact with a concentrated virus (laboratory)	High
Wound or laceration caused by visibly contaminated instruments	Medium
Open wound contamination	Medium
Surface wound	Low
Closed wound contamination	Low
Prolonged contact of large skin portions	Low
Contamination of small portions of intact skin, with blood or wound caused by objects not visibly contaminated	Not shown

Source: PHASE Study, 2003[6]

51

Tab. 3.3 Hygienic and environmental risks

Chemical agents (exposure risks)	- Ingestion - Cutaneous contact - Inhalation of dust, fumes, gases, vapors
Physical agents	- Noisy equipment - Ultrasound - Radiation - Lighting (shortages)
Biological agents	- Involuntary emission (air conditioning system); - Uncontrolled emission (waste disposal plants, handling of infected material in the hospital environment); - Treatment or willful manipulation (use of substances for experimental research in vitro or in location of productive activities such as biotechnologies).

Source: ASL Reggio Emilia, 2008[7]

The most important factors directly related to these types of risk are the following (tab. 3.4):

Tab. 3.4 Risk factors

1) Inadequate technology	equipment, ventilation systems
2) Wrong layout of the facility and/or of the workplace:	isolation of the most risky areas
3) Lack of protection equipment	hands, respiratory tract, face
4) Disinfection and discontinuous decontamination	
5) Non-application of basic hygiene rules:	hand washing, correct management of patient hygiene
6) Periodic disposal of waste	
7) Lack of training and behavior management	

Source: SSR Emilia Romagna, dossier n. 109/2005[8]

Structural and organizational risks. They concern, on the one hand, the damage caused by accidents or injuries suffered by the staff involved in the different work activities, following a traumatic physical contact (electrical, mechanical, etc.);
on the other hand, the risks deriving from the complex relationship between operator and the organization in which he carries out his work.

In particular, structural risks result from a situation of imbalance between person and structure, machine or plant, causing serious damage and even physical impairment (tab. 3.5).

Organizational risks result from significant deficiencies in the system of procedures, rules, division of labor, definition of their functions and responsibilities, by jointly considering human, technological and socio-cultural aspects (tab. 3.6).

Tab. 3.5 Structural Risks

Risks from structural weaknesses	- Height, surface and volume of the structure - Lighting - Floors - Outputs - Underground rooms
Risks from safety faults of machinery and equipment	- Protection of working bodies - Machines with CE mark - Protection of lifting equipment, lifts and elevators - Protection in access to tanks
Risks due to lack of electrical safety	- Project Eligibility - User Suitability - Safe installations in environments at risk of fire or explosion
Risks from fire/explosion	- Presence of flammable material - Presence of flammable material deposits - Fire, ventilation and air exchange systems - Safety signs

Source: Risk Assessment Document, ASL Reggio Emilia, 2008

Tab. 3.6 Organizational risks

Work organization	- Weary working processes - Tasks, functions and responsibilities - Lack of control and monitoring programs - Maintenance of plants and safety equipment - Manual handling of loads
Psychological factors	- Intensity/monotony/repetitiveness of work - Non-participation in decision-making - Complexity of tasks - Lack of motivation
Ergonomic factors	- Knowledge and skills of the staff - Communication and information - Ergonomics equipment

Source: Risk Assessment Document, ASL Reggio Emilia, 2008

3.2 Risk Mapping: identification of critical areas

Risk mapping is a task of analysis, essential for identifying areas of interest, where more frequently risky events could occur. By analyzing clinical, organizational and structural processes, safety of people, documents and information systems, it is possible to determine the nature and level of the existing and potential risks, in order to identify corrective measures necessary to re-balance the system.

This requires the involvement of all clinical and organizational staff, in order to integrate risk information acquired during the critical analysis process of the different areas involved.

Currently, there is no a common system of mapping adverse events at national level, associated with critical areas of work. An attempt in this direction was made first by the company "Rasini Viganò Insurance"[9] and subsequently by "AON Insurance"[10].

Lombardy Region has entrusted them with the task of processing and reviewing the claims of Lombard healthcare system, every year. For this reason it can represent an useful reference model for the whole healthcare system, as it is considered the most extensive mapping program on a national scale.

The last revision dates back to 12/31/2016. A reference sample referring to the periods 1999-2015 and 1999-2016[11] was taken into account, to detect the difference in increase or decrease. The sample consists of all the local Lombard healthcare companies, hospitals, IRCCS and Foundations.

A part of the data collected concerns the areas/units that have produced the most requests for civil damages. In particular, the most frequent events occurred in Orthopedics and Traumatology, First Aid, General Surgery, Obstetrics and Gynecology, as shown in the following table (3.7).

Tab. 3.7 Analysis of the main claims for compensation for Specialties/Services

TYPE OF COMPANY: HOSPITAL			
Risk Unit	N. Events 1999-2015	N. Events 1999-2016	Difference
First Aid or Emergency Room	5.142	5.461	+ 319
Orthopedics and traumatology	4.813	5.070	+ 257
Structure (AO-ASL)	3.838	3.976	+ 138
General surgery	3.320	3.465	+ 145
Obstetrics and Gynecology	3.019	3.204	+ 185
General medicine	1.307	1.365	+ 58
Ophthalmology	1.199	1.269	+ 70
Neurosurgery	979	1.049	+ 70
Otorhinolaryngology, audiology	907	957	+ 50
Psychiatry	658	688	+ 30
Radiology	631	665	+ 34
Dentistry and stomatology	622	639	+ 17
Cardiology	585	613	+ 28
Urology	560	601	+ 41
UNIDENTIFIED	467	507	+ 40
Neurology	377	406	+ 29
Pediatrics	375	387	+ 12
Cardiac Surgery	344	369	+ 25
Plastic surgery	309	316	+ 7
Gastroenterology and digestive endoscopy	306	325	+ 19
Anesthesia service	269	277	+ 8
Vascular surgery	265	278	+ 13
Reanimation and intensive care	229	245	+ 16
Recovery and functional	228	233	+ 5

rehabilitation			
Pneumology, tisiology, respiratory physiopathology	202	213	+11
Transfusion center	194	199	+ 5
Oncology	167	178	+ 11
Maxillofacial surgery	166	181	+ 15
Nephrology	144	148	+ 4
Dermatology	143	147	+ 4
Neonatal pathology	129	134	+ 5

Source: AON, Mappatura dei sinistri SSR (Mapping of claims), Regione Lombardia, 1999-2015, 1999-2016

With this tool, it is also possible to verify the incidence of risk and prevalence of the events through a subdivision by macro areas: surgical, first aid, gynecology and obstetrics, pediatric, psychiatric, medical, unidentified.

The results of the following table and graph refer to the analysis by unit of risk in the Hospital Companies whose claims for compensation are higher than those advanced to the Local Health Authorities (ASL) (tab. 3.8, fig. 3.1).

Tab. 3.8 Areas of Risk and Claims for compensation

	2011	2012	2013	2014	2015	2016
Surgical Area	**935**	**929**	**897**	**861**	**749**	**709**
Emergency Room	265	336	269	244	259	226
Structure	**254**	**211**	**174**	-	-	-
Medical	**293**	**267**	**239**	**219**	**203**	**195**
Obstetrics/Gynecology	189	225	202	199	184	178
Services	**223**	**188**	**146**	**151**	**146**	**165**
Pediatric	47	39	46	63	32	32
Psychiatric	35	51	36	37	31	27
Unidentified	-2	33	46	30	35	115
Intensive Services	25	29	22	26	25	20
Directions-Offices	-4	0	9	14	11	1

Source: reworking data from Report AON Insurance 2011-2016

Fig. 3.1 Claims for compensation

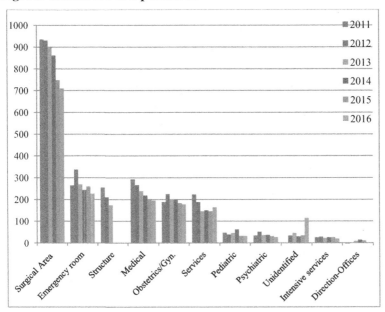

Source: reworking data from Report AON Assicurazioni, 2011-2016

Risk mapping makes it possible to identify critical processes at medium-high risk on which to intervene, determining, at the same time, intervention priorities and actions to improve and contain risks, through the application of reactive and pro-active tools, which will be examined in the next chapters.

3.3 The problem of errors in the exercise of healthcare activity

3.3.1 A classification

The problem of medical errors has been the subject of numerous investigations and studies that have adopted the same approach to analyze and evaluate errors in healthcare.

Based on these analyzes, it was concluded that most of them relate to a system failure (at the organizational level and processes that lead people to make mistakes) and then not only individual factors (due to negligence, incompetence, failure to comply with rules and protocols).

Following the publication of the US Institute of Medicine (IOM), *To err is human, building a safer health system*, the issue of error in medicine has taken on increasing importance at social, institutional and insurance levels.

With it we tried to build a common language, able to give a name to the different types of error, in order to identify root causes of the phenomenon, especially after assessing the extent of the consequences.

From this document it was found that up to 1999:

- every year one million Americans reported damage from medical treatment;
- 98,000 Americans died from medical errors that could be foreseen and avoided;
- about $ 29 billion has been spent for errors and damages (table 3.9).

Furthermore, errors have constantly led to a loss of user confidence in healthcare system and a decrease in satisfaction, both by patients and health professionals (IOM, 1999)[12].

Tab. 3.9 Errors in medicine in the United States

Errors on the total number of patients admitted	3-4%
Preventable errors on the total	53%
Mortality	6,6%
Costs	$ 29 billion

Source: IOM, "To err is human", 1999

"If individual factors represent an important part of clinical practice, however, they constitute an element of a more complex system in which the health worker works. To err is human, accidents can always happen; but it is possible to reduce their frequency by learning from them and implementing defenses able reduce the risk of individual errors"[13].

Starting from a general definition of error, it is possible to identify the various types that most frequently occur in current medical practice. The error represents, always and however, "a failure in planning and/or execution of a sequence of actions that determines the failure to achieve the desired goal, not attributable to the case"[14].

According to James Reason[15], errors can be perceived, on the one hand, as consequences of actions, performed by people who are in direct contact with patients and system (active errors; they can take a variety of profiles as inattention, omissions, oversights, violations);
on the other hand, as the result of decisions taken by management, system planners and procedures, defined by Reason as latent conditions or *"pathogens inborn systems"* which, combined with active errors, are able to create the conditions to break system defenses (tab. 3.10).

Tab. 3.10 Theory of errors (Reason)

Slip	Execution errors occurring at the skill level; the task is performed incorrectly, even knowing the procedures
Lapses	Execution errors caused by a memory failure such as confusion or forgetfulness of planned elements
Mistakes	Applying the wrong rules and procedures (rule-based). Applying the wrong knowledge or lack of knowledge (knowledge-based)
Violations	Actions that are performed not in compliance with regulations or directives

A further and more exhaustive classification is reported in the document issued by the Ministry of Health, *"Risk management in health: the problem of errors"* (2004), which proposes a systemic view of the phenomenon, distinguishing the errors in two categories: general and specific (tab. 3.11).

Tab. 3.11 Types of errors (general and specific errors)

GENERAL ERRORS	
ERRORS OF COMMISSION	Due to the execution of incorrect or undue medical acts
ERRORS OF OMISSION	Due to failure to perform medical records, deemed necessary for the care
HUMAN ERROR	*Slip, lapses, mistakes*
VIOLATIONS	Failure to comply with the procedures
ORGANIZATIONAL ERRORS	Due to work organization, emergency management planning, availability and accessibility of equipment

SPECIFIC ERRORS	
ERROR IN THE USE OF DRUGS	- Prescription - Preparation - Transcription - Distribution/timetable - Administration/dosage - Monitoring
ERROR IN THE MANAGEMENT OF BIOLOGICAL SAMPLES	- Identification/traceability - Methods for sampling, storing and breaking the tubes - Sending and loss of samples
SURGICAL ERROR	- Foreign bodies in the surgical site - Intervention on part or side of the wrong body - Improper surgical execution - Unnecessary surgery - Incorrect treatment of the patient
ERROR IN USE OF EQUIPMENT	- Malfunction due to technical manufacturing problems - Use in improper conditions

	- Inadequate maintenance - Inadequate instructions - Incorrect cleaning - Use beyond the time limits provided
EXAMINATIONS OR DIAGNOSTIC PROCEDURES	- Not performed - Planned but not implemented - Inadequately or incorrectly performed - Not appropriate
ERRORS IN THE TIMING	- Delay in drug treatment - Delays in surgery - Delay in diagnosis - Other organizational, managerial and logistic delays
ERRORS IN DISINFECTION AND STERILIZATION OF PRESIDES AND TOOLS	- No decontamination, incorrect disinfection - Use of non-sterile needles containers - Lack of process indicators, lack of knowledge of procedures

In the healthcare sector, the different types of errors and events can be reclassified according to the following table, as shown in the results of the AON Insurance survey, in the periods 1999-2015 and 1999-2016. Again, it takes into account the claims in hospitals (tab. 3.12).

Tab. 3.12 Claims Analysis by type of events and errors (Hospital)

CLASSIFICATION	Situation as of 31/12/2015 (1999-2015)	Situation as of 31/12/2016 (1999-2016)	Difference
Surgical error	8.658	9.124	+ 466
Diagnostic error	6.928	7.387	+ 459
Fall	2.889	3.019	+ 130
Damage to things	2.426	2.480	+ 54
Therapeutic error	2.612	2.757	+ 145
Infections	1.772	1.888	+ 116
Loss	1.539	1.603	+ 64
Invasive procedures	1.346	1.417	+ 71
Unidentified	1.129	1.236	+ 107
Anesthesiological error	847	883	+ 36
Service level	756	792	+ 36
Damage to people	658	678	+ 20
Injury	618	645	+ 27
Prevention error	509	534	+ 25
Theft	362	372	+ 10
Aggression	262	272	+ 10
Defective material	157	175	+ 18
Auto lesion	97	101	+ 4
Lesion of workers' rights	91	95	+ 4
Defective machinery	91	94	+ 3
Professional disease	56	58	+ 2
TOTAL			

Source: reworking by AON Report: 1999-2015, 1999-2016

3.3.2 Risks of particular gravity: Sentinel Events

The adverse event is any unexpected, preventable and non-preventable event (mistake) that can cause an unintentional harm to the patient. It is called *"sentinel"* because it signals the need for an immediate action and response, due to the extreme gravity of the consequences, such as physical and psychological damage or even death.

The issue was dealt with in a document drawn up by the Ministry of Health (*Protocol for monitoring sentinel events*) which, in addition to providing a precise definition of them, pursues the objective of identifying a common policy for monitoring and managing these events at national level.

In this document sentinel events are defined as "serious adverse events, indicative of a serious malfunction of the system, which cause death or serious damage to the patient and lead to a loss of confidence in the Health Service".

It was borrowed from the JCAHCO document (*Joint Commission on Accreditation of Healthcare Organizations*)[16], which has developed guidelines for identifying, reporting and evaluating sentinel events, implementing strategies to prevent them (*Setting the Standard: The Joint Commission and Health Care Safety and Quality*).

In Italy events being monitored are 16 and are shown below (Sentinel Event Monitoring Protocol, Ministry of Health, 2012)[1]:

1) treatment on the wrong patient;
2) surgical procedure on the wrong part of the body;
3) wrong procedure on correct patient;
4) instruments or other material left inside the surgical site, that requires an additional operation or procedure;

5) transfusion reaction due to incompatibility of A-B-0 groups;
6) death, coma or severe harm resulting from errors in drug therapy;
7) maternal death or serious illness related to labor and/or childbirth;
8) death or permanent disability in a healthy newborn weighing > 2500 g., not related to congenital disease;
9) death or severe damage due to patient fall;
10) suicide or attempted suicide of a patient in a hospital;
11) violence on patient;
12) acts of violence against the operator;
13) death or serious damage resulting from a malfunction of the transport system;
14) death or serious damage resulting from an incorrect assignment of the triage code in the Operations Center 118 and/or within the Emergency Room;
15) death or serious unforeseen damage due to surgery;
16) any other adverse event that causes death or serious harm to the patient.

As mentioned above, the events identified by the Ministry of Health derive from an electronic document published periodically since 1998 on the website of the JCAHO (*Sentinel Event Alert*).

The latter is a non-profit organization engaged in the field of accreditation of healthcare organizations that, since 1995, has started a process of identification of a long series of highly risky events that must be reported by all the structures and accredited institutions, on pain of withdrawal of accreditation itself.

Furthermore, it has the task of identifying possible

solutions to the shortcomings and inefficiencies found and reported, which are the source and cause of these events.

Total number of Sentinel Events reviewed by the Joint Commission from 1995 through 2017 are 13.346. Table 3.13 shows the data on the type, number and incidence of sentinel events, relating to the period 2004-2014, while table 3.14 shows the number of events relating to the years 2015, 2016 and 2017.

Tab. 3.13 Type of Sentinel Event - 2004/2014 (JCAHO)

TYPE OF SENTINEL EVENT	N.
Wrong–patient, wrong-site, wrong-procedure	1.072
Delay in treatment	937
Operative/post-operative complication	823
Suicide	814
Fall	664
Other unanticipated event *	559
Medication error	428
Criminal event	361
Perinatal death/injury	291
Med equipment-related	218
Infection-related event	172
Transfusion error	124
Maternal death	120
Fire	114
Anesthesia-related event	104
Patient elopement	93
Ventilator death	48
Restraint related event	28
Utility system failure	7
Infant abduction	3

Source: JCAHO, 2014, www.jointcommission.org

Tab. 3.14 Type of Sentinel Event (2015, 2016, 2017)

TYPE OF SENTINEL EVENT	2015	2016	2017 partial
Unintended retention of a foreign body	123	120	41
Wrong–patient, wrong-site, wrong-procedure	120	104	35
Delay in treatment	83	54	32
Operative/post-operative complication	82	45	12
Suicide	98	87	43
Fall	95	92	49
Other unanticipated event *	58	47	34
Medication error	47	33	19
Criminal event	47	32	16
Perinatal death/injury	43	23	10
Med equipment-related	14	10	4
Infection-related event	13	2	0
Transfusion error	9	5	2
Maternal death	6	7	3
Fire	26	15	6
Anesthesia-related event	7	4	3
Patient elopement	7	9	3
Ventilator death	3	2	2
Restraint related event	7	7	3
Utility system failure	1	1	0
Infant abduction	3	2	0

Source: Summary Data of Sentinel Events by The Joint Commission, 07/11/2017[18]

Other unanticipated event includes: Asphyxiation, Burn, Choked on food, Drowned, Found unresponsive

On the one hand, most of these events highlight very serious organizational shortcomings of the whole system (including the inadequacy of hospital environments and spaces, problems of relationships and communication within working groups);

on the other hand, an underestimation (by health workers) of important risk factors that lead to delays in treatment and serious therapeutic and care disabilities (unintended retention of a foreign body, wrong–patient, wrong-site, wrong procedure, fall).

The most important problem that arises today is to identify avoidable errors, so that they do not repeat over time; but to realize these objectives it is necessary to investigate the main causes of error and identify effective strategies and tools for preventing and eliminating them.

There is an obligation (especially moral) on the part of healthcare professionals, that is: acting with awareness, responsibility, implementing ethically correct behaviors in the interest of the patient, who represents the most important subject from the point of view of medical assistance.

References

1. ALBERGO F., (2014), *Strumenti di controllo e analisi del rischio nelle aziende sanitarie*, Ed. Cacucci.
2. CONFORTINI M.C., PATRINI E., (2006) *Manuale di risk management in sanità processi e strumenti di implementazione*, Il Sole24 Ore.
3. WORLD HEALTH ORGANIZATION, (2005), *Who draft guidelines for adverse event reporting and learning system*.
4. VINCENT C., ADAMS S.T., STANHOPE N., (1998), *Una cornice di riferimento per l'analisi dei rischi e della sicurezza nella medicina clinica. Original title: Framework for analyzing safety in clinical medicine*, BMJ 1998: 316: 1154-7.
5. ISPEL (1998), *Linee guida per la valutazione del rischio nella piccola e media impresa*.
6. GRUPPO DI STUDIO PHASE, (2001), *Rischio biologico e punture accidentali negli operatori sanitari: un approccio organizzativo e gestionale alla prevenzione in ambito sanitario-ospedaliero*, Milano, Lauri.
7. ASL REGGIO EMILIA, (2008), *Documento di valutazione dei rischi*.
8. SSR EMILIA ROMAGNA, (2005), *Il rischio biologico in "Rischio e sicurezza in sanità"*, dossier n. 109.
9. RASINI VIGANÒ ASSICURAZIONI, (1999-2007), *Mappatura dei sinistri di RCT/O del Sistema Sanitario Regionale Lombardo*.
10. AON Assicurazioni - Risk Management Advisory, (2008-2013), *Mappatura del rischio del sistema sanitario regionale*.

11. AON, *Mappatura dei sinistri SSR* (*Mapping of claims*), Regione Lombardia, 1999-2015, 1999-2016

12. IOM, 1999, Institute Of Medicine, Extract of "To Err Is Human".

13. WRIGHT J., HILL P., (2005), *Clinical Governance*, McGraw-Hill.

14. GLOSSARIO DEL MINISTERO DELLA SALUTE, (2006), *La sicurezza dei pazienti e la gestione del rischio clinico.*

15. REASON J., (2000), *Human error: models and management*, BMJ; 320: 768-770.

16. www.jcaho.org

17. MINISTRY OF HEALTH, (2012), *Protocollo Monitoraggio Eventi Sentinella (Sentinel Events Monitoring Protocol).*

18. JOINT COMMISSION, *Summary Data of Sentinel Events*, 07/11/2017

CHAPTER 4

STRATEGIC PROCESS OF RISK MANAGEMENT

Summary: 4.1 Strategic process. *4.1.1 Why Risk Management in Health Care? 4.1.2 Risk Management steps: using the ERM model in the Healh Care System.* - 4.2 Prevention strategies and risk reduction. *4.2.1 Guidelines and Recommendations* - References

4.1 Strategic process

4.1.1 Why Risk Management in Health Care?

Even in the healthcare system there is a need to foresee and introduce risk management activities and tools to prevent errors that often compromise the quality of care, patient satisfaction and safety of services provided at every level of clinical and organizational system.

However, unlike other organizational and entrepreneurial contexts, the term *safety* refers, on the one hand, to compliance with rules, protocols and regulations that govern structural and technological aspects;
on the other hand, it evokes the concept of *system reliability*, understood as the result of the interaction between organizational, human, cultural and technical factors, in which the state of health and safety of the

person becomes central.

Despite the extraordinary advances in medicine, especially at a technological level, doctors, nurses and other health professionals continue to have a special ethical and moral responsibility in meeting their patients' needs, including maintaining and improving the quality of care they provide[1].

Therefore, it is inevitable that healthcare providers adopt an approach to the problem both administrative (insurance policy management, cost containment and productivity increase), but also aimed at the continuous improvement of clinical practice, patient care and quality, which involves the whole organization and activity.

In the context of risk management, the concept of *governance* cannot be excluded; it presupposes a reorganization and a profound cultural change by all stakeholders in the healthcare system, to ensure a quality management of health services.

According to the most widespread definition, *governance* is "a system and a framework by which National Health Service organizations take account of the continuous improvement of quality of their services and safeguarding of high standards of care, through the creation of a context in which excellence in clinical care must be guaranteed"[2].

Healthcare system is a complex organism formed by different levels (clinical, organizational, contractor, accredited and regional apparatuses) that requires a dynamic and flexible business management, to meet the expectations of all stakeholders.

To achieve this, it is necessary to adopt tools and mechanisms that emphasize principles such as professionalism, competence, patient-to-patient relationship, ability to work in groups and, in particular, self-correcting ability and self-regulation in the exercise of an increasingly heterogeneous and complex activity.

Risk management is an essential element of the governance system, especially if one considers, on one side, the multidimensional aspect of health risk that ranges from pure or clinical risk to non-health risk (administrative, logistical, structural safety, fraud, emergencies);
on the other side, an increased control, safety and quality requirements contribute to the development of management strategies and operating processes.

In this regard, it may be useful to briefly identify and describe the essential features of the other dimensions that help to set up an integrated governance system.

This concept appeared for the first time in the document *"Governing the NHS: a Guide for NHS Boards"* (NHS Commission, 2003), to emphasize the opportunity to integrate the different levels of governance (clinical, managerial, informative, cultural), with the goal of designing an aggregate tool that induces organizational actors to pursue a mission characterized by certain peculiarities, compared to other organizations (fig. 4.1).

Fig. 4.1 *Quality is improved by integrating the different dimensions of a system*

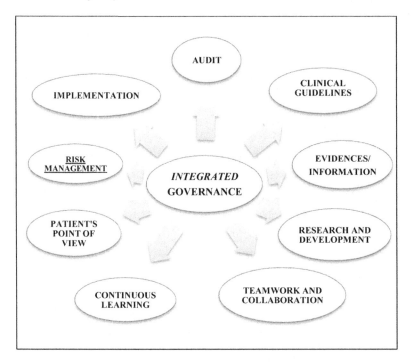

Source: adaptation by Wright, Hill, 2005, p. 48

The elements that support an integrated governance system are as follows (adaptation by Wright-Hill, 2005, p. 46)[2]:

a. **Audit**: it is a technique for identifying critical areas to be reviewed, through the examination of clinical documentation or interviews; it pursues the improvement of health and quality.

b. **Guidelines**: they are recommendations and general protocols aimed at planners and system managers, to improve quality of management and organization.

c. **Clinical Guidelines**: they are recommendations developed in a systematic way to help physicians, patients, to make decisions about the appropriate treatment of specific health conditions.

d. **Evidence/Information**: they are tools to support the guidelines. They are intended to verify effectiveness, reliability and validity of research in the healthcare and clinical trials, through scientific methods, for collecting and analyzing heterogeneous data. For example, in the field of security, one of the most important revisions is the one carried out by *American Agency for Healthcare Research and Quality* in 2001, in the healthcare sector.

e. **Research and Development**: this activity provides for the development of local projects (such as Risk Management), dissemination of innovative practices and practical implementation of research.

f. **Teamwork and Collaboration**: the presence of multidisciplinary teams is essential to ensure high quality performance. In fact, performance depends not only on individual skills but also on the way in which group members interact with each other. For example, it has been shown that in operating rooms, characterized by a high complexity, both from a psychological and organizational point of view, interpersonal and communication problems are often responsible for serious errors and inefficiencies.

g. **Continuous Learning Education and Training**: these are activities that allow constant updating for clinicians and organizations, in order to adapt to changes in the profession.

h. **Patient's Point of View**: involvement and active participation of the patient allow to develop new methodologies to improve clinical practice but also to identify any critical areas (patient reports are an example).

i. **Risk Management**: risk management process is a complex activity, aimed at identifying the most frequent danger situations and instruments for preventing, reducing and eliminating them.
j. **Implementation**: this phase makes it possible to achieve the expected objectives through an integrated and coherent view of all the dimensions analyzed above.

Governance should be considered the primary activity of healthcare organizations to improve the quality of care.

In this context, *Risk Management* becomes an essential element of the system as, both patients and the different health and non-health actors, must be protected from the potential damage caused by the health organization.

Therefore, only through a rigorous design and flexible management of the many quality improvement activities, it is possible to reduce risks, prevent avoidable mistakes and ensure safety. The critical areas, on which to focus for creating a safety culture, are identified in the figure below (fig. 4.2).

Fig. 4.2 The safety culture and context factors behind an effective risk management process

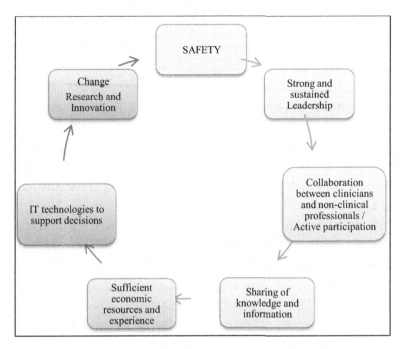

In particular, the presence of a strong leadership, (focused on the continuous improvement of organizational performance and quality of care, supported by an active participation and collaboration between clinical and non-clinical professionals), promotes a change in ethics and culture.

It is aimed at adopting a systemic approach to risk management, which presupposes a conscience and responsibility of all the actors involved in the process, both operationally and strategically.

4.1.2 Risk Management steps: using the ERM model in the Healh Care System

Talking about Risk Management in health means pursuing a business policy oriented to a safety culture, in order to strengthen the awareness and perception of risks (predictable and preventable) that can cause serious patient suffering and economic harm to the business.

It is believed that a risk management system should affect the whole business scope and not just the clinical risk management, relying on the principle of "*promoting and disseminating a risk culture*" among practitioners working in healthcare organizations.

It is the starting point for an effective preventive action, as it is "a systematic process, including both clinical risk management and corporate risk management"; "it employs a set of methods, tools and actions that help to identify, analyze, evaluate and treat risks, in order to improve the safety of patients, staff, visitors and organization in general"[3].

It also includes the "system of guidelines, protocols, pathways, procedures, organizational and clinical practices adopted within a hospital, to reduce the likelihood of events and actions that may potentially produce negative or unexpected effects on the patient health state"[4] and safety of each individual. It is an innovative approach, but above all a countermeasure designed to improve the quality of care, health state and safety in the processes and activities that are most at risk.

As for the Enterprise Risk Management (ERM), it is the need to build a model which includes all the elements required, to effectively manage risk also for healthcare sector (tab. 4.1). In reality, the practical application about techniques used, assessment and control mechanisms, roles and responsibilities assigned, is not achieved according to a strict and absolute set of predefined rules.

This means that every healthcare organization will realize the ERM model according to its own modalities, especially considering the particular complexity of the sector, the culture, management philosophy, specific needs and expectations of the users in question (patients, healthcare professionals, manager).

Tab. 4.1 Elements of the ERM model

INTERNAL ENVIRONMENT
DEFINITION OF OBJECTIVES
IDENTIFICATION OF EVENTS / RISKS
RISK ASSESSMENT
RESPONSE TO RISK
CONTROL ACTIVITY
INFORMATION AND COMMUNICATION
MONITORING

Source: PricewaterhouseCoopers, Il Sole 24 Ore, 2006

The main phases that characterize the health risk management process are (Figure 4.3):
1) identification of the subject to whom to entrust the government of risk management process;
2) identification and analysis of risks;
3) risk assessment;
4) identification of intervention priorities;
5) planning and implementation of intervention procedures;
6) verification and monitoring of all previous phases;
7) communication and consultation.

Fig. 4.3 The process of Health Risk Management

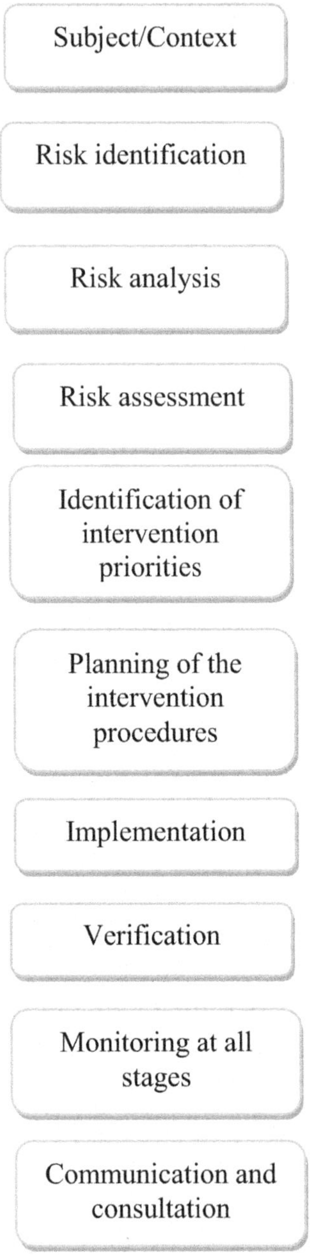

Subject/Context

Risk identification

Risk analysis

Risk assessment

Identification of intervention priorities

Planning of the intervention procedures

Implementation

Verification

Monitoring at all stages

Communication and consultation

Source: adaptation by Report: "Healthcare Risk Management Strategy", HSE Mid Western Area, 2005 [5]

1) Subject/Context. The implementation of an effective risk management program cannot ignore:

a. the presence of an organizational structure suitable to carry out this type of activities;

b. a strong and effective style of leadership that promotes the sharing by all of the strategy that the company intends to achieve; and encourages a real change and a deeper sense of belonging.

In the healthcare practice, risk management activity is assigned to the Risk Management Unit (UGR), coordinated by the risk manager, defined at company level and representative of all the areas involved (clinical, management, legal ones).

This body "must be placed in staff to the General Management of health organizations, must be extended to the network throughout the organization and have a direct and complementary relationship to staff and network for quality.

The team must be coordinated by a medical or health manager with a specific training on the planning, organization and evaluation of health systems oriented to quality and safety, making use of all professional skills and competences available in the organization"[6].

Risk management activity is carried out in collaboration with the Claims Assessment Committee, which has the specific function of managing and assessing incidents and adverse events, coordinated by the Head of General and Legal Affairs.

In some healthcare organizations, such as the Tuscan one, there is the Corporate Committee for Patient Safety which performs advisory and address functions (and which includes the heads of the department or operating units, fig. 4.4).

Fig. 4.4 Structure of Corporate Risk Management

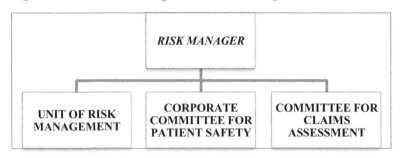

Risk Management Unit, responsible for defining and implementing the business plan, must be composed of professionals belonging to both clinical and managerial/administrative areas (Figure 4.5). The Claims Assessment Committee will also be characterized by the presence of different persons (Figure 4.6)[7].

Fig. 4.5 Structure of the Risk Management Unit

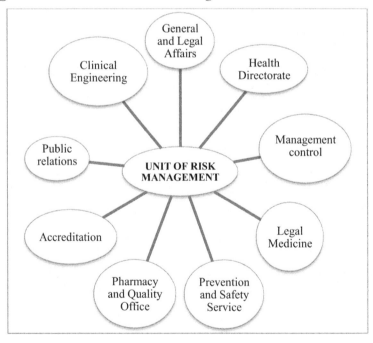

Source: adaptation by Confortini, Patrini, Il Sole 24 Ore, 2006

Fig. 4.6 Structure of Committee For Claims Assessment

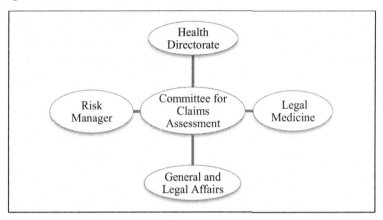

Source: adaptation by Confortini, Patrini, Il Sole 24 Ore, 2006

The functions and activities carried out by this body are complex in nature, because of the strategic role played, within the planning and coordination, for a better realization of the goals set (tab. 4.2).

Tab. 4.2   Activities and functions of the URM

ACTIVITIES	FUNCTIONS
1) Defining tools to identify risks	1) Promoting the culture of risk, sensitizing the operators through continuous training activities
2) Identifying latent critical area	2) Promoting meetings and discussion on what to do
3) Identifying tools to reduce damage to people and structure	3) Evaluating critical areas to contain the negative effects of risks
4) Defining image and communication strategies with users	4) Monitoring the results achieved at each stage of the process
5) Organizing and supporting staff working on the problem	
6) Containing the economic consequences of legal actions	
7) Ensuring that the changes are introduced and evaluated and that the success achieved is enhanced	

Source: adaptation by Confortini, Patrini, Il Sole 24 Ore, 2006; Ovretveit in Siquas, Recommendations on clinical risk management, 2006

2) Identification and analysis risks. The purpose of this step is to identify all the potential risks which are likely to cause losses and decrease in value, with regard to the various corporate resources, through the examination of administrative and clinical data (such as analysis of medical records, complaints or voluntary collection of cards for reporting errors or potential errors by health professionals, *Incident Report*, fig. 4.7).

Fig. 4.7 Sources for risk identification

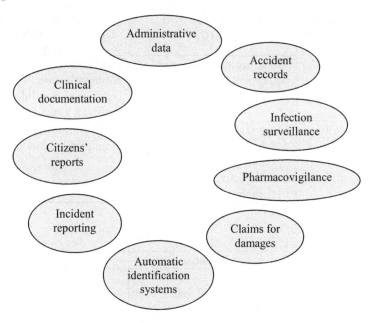

Source: Regional Health Agency Emilia Romagna, Dossier 223-2012[8]

On the other hand, risk analysis allows to search for sources and potential causes of damage, errors and the whole process that has determined them (organizational and management factors, environmental factors, patient-related factors, human factors). It examines what happened and why it happened, identifying for each factor all the conditions that potentially have contributed to the occurrence of accident (tab. 4.3).

Tab. 4.3 Contributing factors

HUMAN FACTORS	ORGANIZATIONAL FACTORS	INTER-ORGANIZATIONAL FACTORS
Slipses	Problems in the design of equipment and technologies	Insufficient communication between stakeholders involved in the event
Mistakes	Environmental and context conditions that discourage operators from reporting incidents and learning from experience	Lack of information among stakeholders
Lapses	Mental and physical conditions that lead to improper performance	
Violations	Shortage of personnel	
Diagnosis errors	- Inadequate training - Lack of control and support procedures - Rigid work distribution - Inappropriate protocols and regulations - Lack of communication and coordination between staff or between departments	

Source: adaptation by Confortini, Patrini, Il Sole 24 Ore, 2006

After identifying the contributing factors that led to the adverse event, it is possible to proceed to the analysis of the *"Root Causes"*, through a series of methods and techniques useful for:

a. monitoring the risks of the activities and services underlying them;

b. identifying the causes.

The methods and techniques of risk management are describes below (Lighter D.E, 2011)[9]:

1) Methods:
- **RCA** (*Root Cause Analysis*): it is a problem-solving process that investigates events of particular interest. It focuses not so much on the search for individual responsibilities, but on why it happened and on the actions to be taken to prevent repetition.
- **FMEA** (*Failure Mode and Effect Analysis*)**:** it is a qualitative and forecasting method in which all the possible ways of error or failure, their effects and potential causes are listed. Based on judgments provided by experts, it allows to identify the weak points of a process or a project and to eliminate the identified faults, modifying the process/project itself.
- **FMECA** (*Failure Mode, Effect and Criticality Analysis*): it is a method that is always predictive, but compared with the previous one, it uses quantitative data, estimating for each event the severity, probability and relevance.
- **HFMEA** (*Healthcare Failure Mode and effect Analysis*): this method was introduced by the National Center for Patient Safety, in collaboration with the Department of Veteran Affaire for application in healthcare. Through a worksheet, everything that is done during the survey is summarized, from the analysis of risks and dangers, to the actions taken and results achieved
- **CREA** (*Clinical Risk and Error Analysis*): it is a quantitative method; it uses statistical literature studies that elaborate error historical data on different treatment processes.

2) Techniques used:
- **Asking why? The Five-Why**: it is a technique used in the RCA to investigate the causes of each level, proceeding to identify the most remote cause of the problem in question.

- **Fishbone diagram**: it is used to represent all the possible causes, classifying them and grouping the contributing factors by default.
- **Event card and causal factors**: it shows the relationships between events and their causal factors using a logical sequence, identifying where and when errors occurred in the sequence of events.
- **Hazard barrier target analysis**: it analyzes three aspects: the risk, the barrier and the target. It is used to plan corrective actions.
- **Check list**: it is based on the classification of the causes that, through a series of questions, guides the analysis activity (What happened? Why it happened? What are the next factors?).

The following example concerns the analysis of an adverse event in the orthopedic and traumatological field, by reviewing medical records (Figure 4.8). It turns out that "an insufficient completeness of the medical record makes inevitable the underestimation of the adverse events, affecting the validity of the results, so as to induce erroneous evaluations on their identification and predictability"[10].

Fig. 4.8 Example of analysis of an adverse event

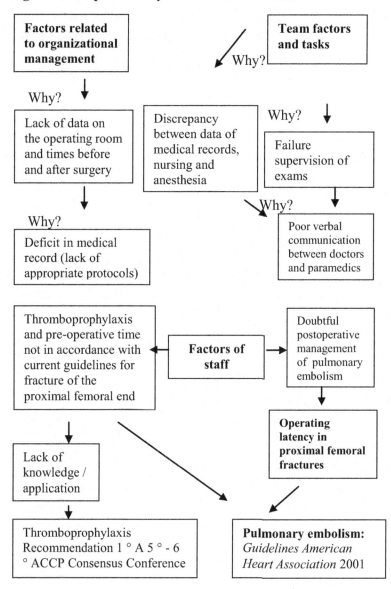

Source: Cuzzupoli, Soccetti, Catalani, De Palma, Clinical risk in proximal femoral fractures, G.I.O.T. 2005; 31: 90-5

3) Risk assessment. As in the ERM model, also in the health risk management process the level of risk can be estimated through qualitative techniques (judgment and experience of health personnel) and quantitative ones (probabilistic data of recurrence of the error and the possible consequent damage). Evaluation can be performed for individual tasks, activities and processes, depending on the complexity of the problem to be analyzed. In the case of quantitative evaluation, a table is prepared and it contains all the elements identifying the process (tab. 4.4).

Tab. 4.4 Quantitative assessment

Code	Description of the activity	Dangerous situations	Code	Ways of potential errors	Probability of error	Severity of damage	Risk

Subsequently, through the risk assessment matrix, the degree of priority of intervention is determined on specific dangerous tasks, activities or parts of process (tab. 4.5).

Tab. 4.5 Assessment matrix of quantitative risk

	No damage	Light damage	Average damage	Serious damage	Death
Frequent					
Probable					
Occasional					
Remote					

Source: Ministry of Health, Risk Management in Healthcare. The problem of errors, 2004.

☐ Acceptable risk: monitoring interventions
☐ Low risk: programming interventions
☐ Medium risk: urgent action
■ High risk: emergency interventions

Qualitative assessment is performed using the damage severity and estimate of probability of occurrence (tables 4.6, 4.7).

Tab. 4.6 Qualitative assessment - Estimation of damage severity

LEVEL OF DAMAGE	DESCRIPTION
No damage	- The error did not involve any damage or made it necessary to monitor the patient - No damage occurred to the service or organization - The economic-financial implications are irrelevant
Slight	- The error has caused temporary damage to the patient and has made or has resulted in a longer hospital stay. - The impact could threaten the efficiency of some aspects of the organization - Some economic-financial implications
Middle	- The error has caused temporary disability to the patient resulting in prolonged hospital stay - The impact could threaten the efficiency of the whole organization - Modest economic-financial implications
Serious	- The error caused permanent disability or next event involved a death, such as anaphylactic shock and cardiac arrest - Serious implications for the organization's efficiency and for economic and financial aspects
Catastrophic	- Patient's death - Organization unable to carry out its functions - Very serious economic and financial implications

Source: adaptation by NHS, *Risk Management Strategy*, 2006[11]; Ministry of Health, Risk Management in Healthcare. The problem of errors, 2004

Tab. 4.7 Qualitative assessment-Estimated probability of occurrence (expressed as number of errors per 100 admissions)

Probability of occurrence of the error	Probability range
Remote	Less then 0,3%
Occasional	0,3% – 7%
Probable	7% - 14%
Frequent	More then 14%

Source: Ministry of Health, Risk Management in Healthcare. The problem of errors, 2004

4) Identification of intervention priorities. As part of this activity, the goal is to identify areas in which, more frequently, dangerous situations could emerge, distinguishing the strictly clinical area from organizational and structural ones.

For example, in the event that the potential incident occurs due to a lack of communication between staff or dissemination of incorrect information, the factors to be analyzed and assessed are not only those attributable to the individual's responsibility.

They concern, above all, factors relating to the conditions in which the work was carried out, as well as to the characteristics of leadership, which proved to be weak in spreading the culture of collaboration and involvement of the persons concerned (Individual - Organization - System).

5) Planning of intervention programs. When the area in which the most critical situations occur is identified (work organization in the operating room or in the departments, inadequate training of some operators, lack of communication, etc.), it is essential to proceed with the planning and implementation of reliable tools to rebalance, reduce or eliminate negative effects of the damage caused.

If the critical area is communication, staff should be sensitized through involvement in training activities, in order to enhance and improve the following strategic aspects (Ovreitveit, 2005)[12]:
- verbal and written communication;
- communication between young staff and the elderly;
- communication between professions, between specialties and departments;
- appropriate deliveries between shifts;
- availability of the required documentation;
- search for supervision and help;
- availability and responsiveness of older staff;
- the will of the youngest to be helped;
- clear definition of responsibilities;
- teamwork;
- balance in the staff between young and old between doctors and nurses.

6) Verification and monitoring of all the previous phases. This phase involves the activation of regular and constant monitoring and feedback systems, to verify the effect of the measures undertaken at each level of the risk management process, in order to start, where necessary, any further improvement actions.

In fact, the management process is dynamic; the risks change as well as the resources available and the tools used by the company to face the risk. Therefore, the UGR will be to periodically review effectiveness of the actions undertaken, formulate new targets for risk reduction and monitor over time the evolution of risks and Risk Management program[13].

7) Communication and consultation. At every stage of risk management process, every action taken must be

95

communicated by the responsible parties to the interested parties (top management and staff), in order to communicate and acquire useful information to assess the consequences of risk and to reduce/eliminate the sources of risk detected. The change that will follow will have to take place in a systematic and planned manner, since it will concern the integration of Risk Management with the whole quality management system and human resources.

4.2 Prevention strategies and risk reduction

In the healthcare sector, identifying a general strategy of risk reduction and elimination means, first of all, promoting specific actions and interventions to change attitudes, procedures, systems and organizational culture, according to a continuous, safety-oriented improvement approach. In fact, the greatest risks are those attributable to a series of organizational conditions, rarely verifiable by those who actually make the mistake[14]. The analysis of these conditions brings out a set of dysfunctions, related to every level of the structure (person-system, doctor-patient, healthcare professionals-managerial ones).

According to L. Leape[15], in every organization, oriented to safety, risk reduction requires a substantial and sustained commitment by all levels of the system, where each individual recognizes and accepts a personal responsibility to identify and report situations of uncertainty and danger, in order to facilitate their elimination.

He also states that prevention and error reduction strategies exclude highly inspection and sanctioning systems (which certainly do not facilitate explanation of the error) and lead to an increase in incident reporting from 10 to 20%. In this context, Leape identifies some fixed and essential points for the development of an effective strategy:

- the need for a strong leadership, in the absence of which any attempt at improvement would be useless;
- supporting the shift from a punitive system, which causes personal distress and error concealment, to a non-punitive system (provided that the error is not caused by negligence or misconduct);
- a redesign of the responsibilities that lead individuals to perform their functions with care, competence and conscientiousness.

Still Leape states: "but they will still make errors. Who is responsible? The organizations and systems. Who is responsible for the systems? Managers.

Consider a nurse who makes a serious medication dose error. If one of the factors leading her to make the error is that she is working a second shift, or has a doubled patient load, or is inadequately trained for her responsibilities, whose responsibility is that?

Of course, if a doctor or nurse has injured a patient through an error caused by egregious misconduct, neglect, or criminal activity, he or she must be punished. But if such a person had a prior history of reckless behavior and disregard of safe practices, why has he or she been permitted to continue working?

Simply put, management must manage for patient safety just as they manage for efficiency and profit maximization. And safety must become part of what a hospital or health care organization prides itself on".

The main objective is to find the right tools to understand

the root of the problem, since many errors are, in most cases, committed by a person, considered to be the last link in a chain that begins with management decisions, often little addressed to quality and safety policies and to a system of clear and non-conflictual rules.

It is necessary to support and promote the value and benefits of a safety culture (an indispensable pre-requisite of an effective risk prevention and elimination strategy), involving all the interested stakeholders (patients, clinicians, managers), also by defining new rules and procedures that suggest methods for learning where, when, why and how mistakes occur and how to respond to them[16].

4.2.1 Guidelines and Recommendations

In this context, the guidelines represent a point of reference not only for operational clinical practice, but also for management practice. In fact, they are written recommendations of clinical-organizational behavior that propose a set of indications, aimed at supporting the decision-making process of doctors (about treatment processes) and managers (about management processes).

They can also be used by the same patients to be more aware and to participate more actively in health care that concern them.

The most important reason for using guidelines is to improve management, safety and patient care models. To be really useful and effective "they must be scientifically valid, properly developed, disseminated and put into practice"[2].

The goals they intend to pursue are[17]:

- produce useful information to direct the decisions of operators (clinical or otherwise), towards a greater effectiveness, appropriateness and an increased efficiency in the use of resources;

98

- make information easily accessible;
- examine the optimal conditions for introduction into practice;
- evaluate organizational and result impacts.

The expected results concern different categories:

- <u>users</u>, who have the opportunity to be more informed and aware of scientific reasoning in support of the previous treatments;
- <u>healthcare organizations</u>, which can define and optimize care processes and plan their investments;
- the different <u>levels of government</u> (State, Regions, Health authorities), which can reduce inequality in the allocation of services, through programming processes and facilitate monitoring of the quality of services provided;
- <u>professionals</u>, who have in the guidelines a tool for education and improvement of the relationship with patients and a protection for medico-legal risks[17].

The elements that configure the guidelines are described in the following table (tab. 4.8).

Tab. 4.8 Characteristics of the Guidelines

Choice of topic	The guidelines may concern different management and assistance aspects; it is important to evaluate the consequences on the organization and on patients in terms of: 1) costs for health services; 2) risk for life or for health and safety conditions
Identification of strengths and weaknesses	It is necessary to consider: 1) the availability of human and economic resources; 2) support from the hospital; 3) lack of knowledge and skills of the personnel involved
Creation of a work group	Formation of a representative multi disciplinary group in the professionals involved in the application of guidelines
Identification of the necessary changes	There are factors that facilitate and hinder change. The latter can be: 1) structural and organizational ones; 2) linked to established habits among the same operators; 3) individual factors related to knowledge and attitudes; 4) factors related to the doctor-patient relationship related to communication shortcomings or patient expectations. The strategies to promote change are: a) interventions on individual operator (training programs or distribution of information cards); b) structural and organizational interventions (revision of roles and professional skills for problem management, introduction of new technologies, changing of diagnostic-therapeutic pathways).
Preparation of people and context	It is necessary that all operators take a positive attitude and have the required skills

Identification of the work program	It is important to identify the topic to be treated and the time it is expected to use.
Identification of the evidence arising from research	The tests may include clinical trials, case studies, expert opinions or expert committees.
Collective and coordinated actions	Everyone must agree on the objectives to be achieved and on the deadlines identified for the actions planned along the route.
Making the Guidelines accessible	The guidelines must represent documents that are quick and easy to consult, useful for both physicians and patients.
Evaluation of progress	Performing continuous monitoring of the procedure
Update	Integrating the document with any new information, by changing or adding the monitoring indicators

Source: adaptation by Istituto Superiore della Sanità, Agenzia per i Servizi Sanitari Regionali, 2004 and Wright J., Hill P., 2005.

The guidelines, based on the recommendations, derive from the existing literature and systematic reviews, from the concordant opinion of experts at national and international level. Recommendations can be general or specific.

In the first case, they are directed to the whole healthcare organization and may concern statements on the leadership to be taken, to ensure safety; the promotion of a culture of security; the improvement of training interventions and reporting systems (a) (tab. 4.9).

In the second case, the recommended specific actions are related to a process or to a particular activity.

Examples of this are the recommendations on clinical risk management, issued by the Society for Quality in Health Care (b) and those issued by the Ministry of Health, about removal of potassium chloride from the inpatient wards, the adoption of the code bars for drugs or blood products and those related to the prevention of transfusion reaction (c).

Tab. 4.9 Examples of recommendations

(a) General recommendations	(Recommendations from the Canadian review on hospital safety interventions (Wong & Beglaryan, 2004 in Ovreitveit, 2005)[12]
(b) Specific recommendations (Process)	Recommendations on clinical risk management for patient safety, 2006 (SIQuAS – Società Italiana per la Qualità dell' Assistenza Sanitaria)
(c) Specific recommendations (Activities)	Recommendation for prevention of transfusion reaction to the incompatibility of groups A- B – O, (Ministero della Salute, 03/2007)

Guidelines come as a tools (they are a set of interdependent recommendations) for defining welfare and organizational strategies, with the aim to minimize the uncertainty of decisions to be taken in the healthcare context.

The application of these documents will produce real changes only in the presence of strategies that take into account the particular organizational and management characteristics of the local contexts and working conditions.

References

1. LYNN, J., M.A. BAILY, M. BOTTRELL et al., (2007), *The Ethics of Using Quality Improvement Methods in Health Care*, Annals of Internal Medicine; 146 (9):666-673.

2. WRIGHT J., HILL P., (2005), *La Governance clinica*, McGraw-Hill.

3. GLOSSARIO DEL MINISTERO DELLA SALUTE, (2006), *La sicurezza dei pazienti e la gestione del rischio clinico.*

4. ELEFANTI M. IN CINEAS, (2002), *Quando l'errore entra in ospedale.*

5. HSE MID WESTERN AREA, (2005), *Healthcare Risk Management Strategy* Report.

6. SIQUAS, Società Italiana per la Qualità dell'Assistenza Sanitaria, (2006), *Raccomandazione 3.*

7. CONFORTINI M.C.- PATRINI E., (2006), *Manuale di risk management in sanità processi e strumenti di implementazione*, Il Sole24 Ore.

8. AGENZIA REGIONALE SANITARIA EMILIA ROMAGNA, (2012), *Analisi e Misurazione dei Rischi nelle Organizzazioni Sanitarie*, Dossier n. 223.

9. LIGHTER D.E, (2011), *Advanced Performance Improvement in Health Care* by Jones and Bartlett Publisher.

10. CUZZUPOLI P., SOCCETTI A., CATALANI A., DE PALMA L., (2005), *Rischio clinico nelle fratture prossimali di femore.* G.I.O.T; 31: 90-5.

11. NHS LITIGATION AUTHORITY, (2006), *Risk Management Strategy NO.RM01.*

12. OVREITVEIT J., (2005), *Quali interventi sono efficaci per migliorare la sicurezza dei pazienti?* Karoliska

Institutet - Centro per il Management Sanitario, Agosto 2005.

13. OSPEDALE DI LECCO, (2004), *Progetto di sviluppo del sistema di Risk Management*.

14. MARCON G., (2003), *Gestione del rischio clinico*, Care 4.

15. LEAPE L.L., (2000), *Can we make health care safe? In Reducing Medical Errors and Improving Patient Safety* - Accelerating Change Today A.C.T. for America's Health, Feb. 2000.

16. BOSK C.L., (2005), *Continuity and Change in the Study of Medical Error - The Culture of Safety on the Shop Floor*, Paper n. 20, Feb. 2005.

17. ISTITUTO SUPERIORE DELLA SANITÀ, Agenzia per i Servizi Sanitari Regionali, CEVEAS, (2004), *Manuale metodologico, Come produrre, diffondere, aggiornare raccomandazioni per la pratica clinica*, Editore ZADIG, aggiornamento Maggio.

CHAPTER 5

OPERATIONAL INSTRUMENTS
FOR RISK MANAGEMENT

Summary: 5.1 Risk identification tools *5.1.1 Incident Reporting 5.1.2 Reporting by Users 5.1.3 Civic Audit* - 5.2 Towards a reactive and proactive risk analysis *5.2.1 Root Cause Analysis 5.2.2 FMEA (Failure Mode and Effect Analysis) and FMECA (Failure Mode, Effect and Criticality Analysis* - 5.3 Risk treatment tools *5.3.1 The use of innovative computerized technologies to improve security and safety. 5.3.2 Case Study: San Raffaele Hospital, Milan.*

5.1 Risk identification tools

5.1.1 Incident Reporting

In the process of improving the quality of care and safety of individuals and health care organizations, the most critical aspect is represented by the difficulty of identifying and using effective models to analyze risks and errors and to prevent them from recurring over time; hence the need to adopt risk identification tools and reactive and proactive analysis tools.

The first ones pursue the aim of collecting information relating to significant events, potentially and truly dangerous, through mandatory or voluntary reporting, in order to improve safety for the patient, healthcare workers and organization in general.

The second ones are directed to research the root causes of occurrence of these events.

With regard to risk identification tools, Incident Reporting is one of the most effective ways to report (spontaneously and voluntarily) adverse events.

It is used for long-term factors, through structured collection and the study of even rare events, in order to provide a basis of analysis for the planning of strategies and corrective actions and to prevent its occurrence in the future.

In the healthcare sector it was used for the first time in 1978 (anesthesia area) by Cooper, who used a technique created to analyze accidents in the aeronautical sector, with the aim of producing a complete database of events[1].

The process of creating a reporting system has been described in a document published by the World Health Organization, which outlines the components and characteristics. It has been adopted by different healthcare systems, including those of Denmark, England, Norway, Ireland, Slovenia and Sweden (adaptation by WHO[2], p. 19, p. 51).

The components and the features of the Reporting process are described below:

1) COMPONENTS.
a) Subject matter of the report (What). In this phase the different types of events to be reported are identified:

- Adverse event: it is a damage caused to the patient, related to the treatment process not always caused by an error (e.g. anaphylactic shock);

- Error: it is a failure in the planning and execution of a series of actions that compromise the achievement of objectives (error of attention, memory, judgment, omission);

- Near miss or event avoided: it is a mistake that has the

potential to cause an adverse event but that does not occur, because it has been intercepted or because it has no consequences for the patient (exchange of drugs instantly recognized);

-<u>Risks and dangerous conditions:</u> they are threats to safety, due to unsafe practices and processes (management, medical equipment.

b) Subject of the report (Who). The reporting system must specify who reports the events. Could be:
- the doctor
- the nurse
- the patient
- the visitor or family members.

c) Report methods (How). It describes the ways in which the event can or should be reported. It depends on the local infrastructures and available technologies:
- reporting cards
- telephone/fax
- Internet/mail.

2) FEATURES OF THE REPORTING PROCESS.

a) Not punitive: the signalers must be free from fear of retaliation or punishment.

b) Confidential: it is possible to make anonymous reported events by eliminating the recognizable elements.

c) Independent: reporting system must be independent of the authorities with the power to punish the signalman or the organization, with a focus on results obtained.

d) Timely: identified events must be reported without delay through, for example, regular publication.

e) System oriented: the recommendations should focus on changes in the system, processes and individual behavior, in order to spread a culture of voluntary reporting.

Incident Reporting aims to make staff aware of any type of event, potentially able to cause harm to the person and organization, for the design of corrective measures related to organizational and individual context in which events occur. In this regard, it is possible to determine the major strengths and weaknesses of this technique (tab. 5.1):

Tab. 5.1 Strengths and Weaknesses

Strengths	Weaknesses
Allows you to report serious or insignificant events (frequent and infrequent)	Subjectivity and discretion in assessing the severity or otherwise of the event (different perception in recognizing an adverse event or near miss)
It allows to identify the causes of the event promptly and to act accordingly	Discretion in reporting
It can prevent the recurrence of similar events in the future	Fear that the report will be used for any disciplinary action or to discredit colleagues
	Fear that the planned corrective actions are not implemented

Source: adaptation by Perrella G., Leggeri R., (2007), *La gestione del rischio clinico,* Franco Angeli Ed.

Alongside the mandatory systems, such as those relating to sentinel events (set up by the Joint Commission)[3], most healthcare organizations have adopted voluntary reporting systems, which consider not only the most serious events but also those whose consequences may be minimal or irrelevant.

In healthcare and internationally, the most significant system is the Australian Incident Monitoring System, introduced in 1996 in Australia in some organizations. Subsequently, it was applied in all operating units of its healthcare system, which are inspired by various Italian healthcare organizations.

The tool used for reporting is a generic card, in which are reported the events (serious, near miss or both) subsequently inserted into a monitoring database for the study of causes of the event.

It can be implemented in the overall structure or in some parts of it (departments, operational units, individual process or activity). In particular, the following table (5.2) shows some examples of events, often reported in medical practice (near miss are distinguished from adverse events).

Tab. 5.2 Types of events (adverse events and near miss)

ADVERSE EVENTS REPORTED	DESCRIPTION
Fall	Patient fell while he was waiting for the glycemic curve
Inaccuracy of therapeutic procedure	Gauze forgotten at the surgical site (feedback at discharge)
Inaccuracy of surgical procedure	Postpartum hemorrhage from bleeding laceration
Inaccuracy of medication	1) Administration of drug at wrong dosage (under dosage); 2) Administration of antibiotic to a patient with intolerance
Omission of welfare services	Failure to make a home pickup, due to difficulty in finding the house of the patient
Failure diagnostic procedure	Non-routine electrocardiogram at the entrance (found for hypotensive episode)
Delay of welfare performance	Not timely replacement of hypotensive patch
Delay of surgical procedure	Delay for general indication of the type of anesthesia
Damage due to bad positioning of the devices	Phlebitis by incorrect positioning of the venous catheter
Hospital infection	Contaminated food

NEAR MISS REPORTED	DESCRIPTION
Inaccuracy of the patient	1) Pick the wrong patient intercepted 2) Exchange of the pre-deposited blood request - Intercepted 3) Transcription of glycemic value on the card of another patient - Intercepted
Inaccuracy of diagnostic procedure	Radiological survey already performed and documented in the medical record
Inaccuracy of the drug	1) Preparation of the wrong drug (another drug) - Intercepted 2) Delivery of the wrong medication to the patient before administration
Omission of welfare services	Risk of failure to perform the blood draw at home, for lack of a suitable test tube
Omission of drug administration	Difficulty to withdraw a drug for reducing the activity of pharmaceutical service (strike)
Delay of surgical procedure	At the time of surgery there was no clinical documentation (examinations not performed before, but done at the time)

Source: adaptation by Agenzia Sanitaria Regionale, Regione Emilia, Dossier 86/2003

After identifying events and causes, the data are reprocessed by the business units involved, to promote corrective actions and the most suitable organizational solutions to be applied to the most critical areas (training, communication, skills, procedures, protocols, technologies, safety mechanisms).

To ensure this goal, it is necessary to present the collected data and results achieved by the personnel involved, to further encourage it in the practice of spontaneous event reporting.

In some foreign healthcare systems, such as the

Australian and American ones, information is also disseminated through publications and newsletters accessible to the public, eliminating personal data related to the patients involved.

5.1.2 Reporting by Users

This system (used by most of the healthcare organizations, in which the ORP - Public Relations Office - was set up) is an active communication technique with citizens. It allows to identify any critical areas of health and organizational dissatisfaction, through the information collected.

The goal is to guide company decisions to the adoption of strategies for improving services and enhancing overall context.

The reports can take the form of complaints, remarks, praises or suggestions (Figure 5.1) and having as their object the following areas[4]:

- structural aspects;
- organizational and bureaucratic aspects;
- technical and professional aspects;
- economic aspects;
- hospitality and comfort aspects;
- information and waiting times.

Fig. 5.1 Types of User Reports and Reports used by Public Relations Offices

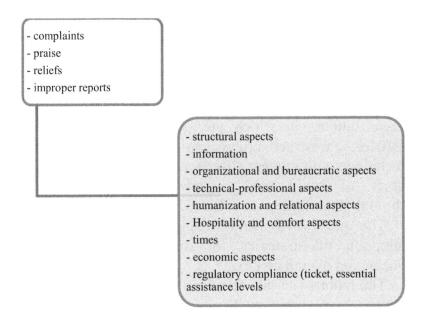

Source: Agenzia Sanitaria Regionale Emilia Romagna, Dossier n. 245/2014[4]

In healthcare risk management, complaints are the most common form for detecting incident events, especially in the areas related to the opportunity/adequacy of services, performance and quality of relational and communication aspects. Interesting in this regard is the analysis carried out by the Emilia Romagna Region, about reports received in 2013 (tab. 5.3).

Tab. 5.3 Reporting Hospitals / Local Health

Complaints	8.298
Praise	9.497
Reliefs	3.047
Suggestions	431
Improper reports	496
Total	**21.769**

Source: Agenzia Sanitaria Regionale Emilia Romagna, Dossier n. 245/2014[4]

This type of system pursues the aim of creating a continuous feedback between company and citizen, in order to verify how quality is perceived in the different organizational areas, planning improvement actions and improving the ability to distinguish reports of interest for risk management.

5.1.3 Civic Audit[5]

It is an initiative that comes from the collaboration of representatives and heads of the *Court of the Sick People Rights - Cittadinanzattiva*, certification bodies, operators and experts of the Health Authorities, as a tool for assessing healthcare structures, to deal with three types of problems:
1) representing the citizens' point of view;
2) to make transparent and verifiable the action of Health Authorities;
3) to prevent the risk of an excessive fragmentation, due to the presence of different systems, for the rights protection and benefits provision.

Through direct observation, the request for information about current status of the structures involved, consultation of administrative documents and examination of citizens' reports, a comparison is made of company performance:

- to identify a set of homogeneous and shared indicators;
- to highlight important critical areas and encourage the adoption of corrective actions.

Among the areas and interventions under evaluation, are included those related to risk management, at company level and hospital care. Some of the improvement actions, undertaken by companies, are as follows:

- actions on structures;
- organizational adjustments;
- launch of projects (including Risk Management), with the production of guidelines and establishment of multidisciplinary teams;
- implementation of actions through collection points, for complaints and logistics and healthcare information;
- implementation of communication via a website.

Generally, the indicators and elements used, to assess the level and results achieved by the Health companies involved in Audit projects, are:

- Office/person in charge of management, at any level of the structure;
- recording of errors, almost errors, accidents deriving from organizational problems, sentinel events;
- drawing up a risk map;
- preparation of a risk management plan;
- Commission for the prevention of hospital infections;
- Committee for the good use of blood;
- specific training courses on risk management;

- Commission for the drafting of guidelines or formal adoption of guidelines drawn up at regional or national level;
- procedures for maintaining constant relations between administrative sector and departments in managing disputes.

In healthcare practice, Audit has proved to be an effective tool for the critical analysis of emerged situations and systematic application of strategies, to improve quality of services and services provided.

In most of the assessed structures, this has been achieved through the interaction between actors (health and non-health), engaged in a constant monitoring of the results achieved.

5.2 Towards a reactive and proactive risk analysis

5.2.1 Root Cause Analysis (RCA)

The identification of events is necessary because, with the data coming from Incident Reporting, it is possible on the one hand, to investigate proximal causes or contributing factors to the event, reconstructing the sequence of events (reactive analysis: RCA);
on the other hand, highlight the vulnerability of processes and system, avoiding adverse events, potentially dangerous for the person and organizational structure (proactive analysis: FMEA/FMECA, 5.2.2).

RCA is "a retrospective analysis that allows to understand what, how and why an event happened. It can be applied in all healthcare settings and requires to investigate areas such as communication, staff training and experience, work planning, local procedures, environment and equipment, barriers"[6].

The goal is to go back to the most remote *root causes* of the event, reconstructing the sequence of events. It focuses not so much on the search for the *"culprit"*, but on the failure of the system, processes and activities.

The Reason model traces the root causes in terms of organization and work environment, analyzing the interaction and concatenation between different and potential causal factors[7] (fig. 5.2).

Fig. 5.2 Reason's Model

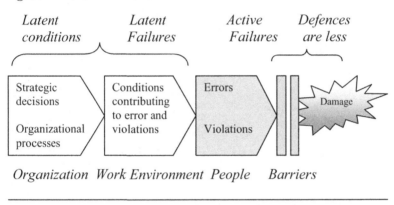

Source: adaptation by Reason,1996, ASR Emilia Romagna, Dossier 130/06

The way in which RCA takes place involves a coordinated process of actions, aimed at a classification and description of events (What happened?) and causes identification (Why did it happen?) (fig. 5.3).

Fig. 5.3 Root Cause Analysis process (RCA)

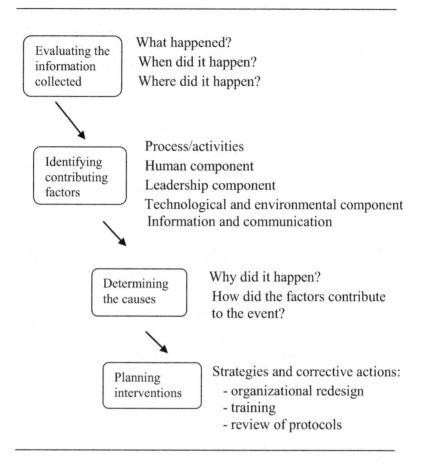

Source: adaptation by ASR Emilia Romagna, Dossier 130-2006, Confortini-Patrini, Il Sole 24 Ore, 2006[8]

It is divided into a series of phases or logical steps, necessary to ensure effectiveness and to identify priority cases to be analyzed:

1) *indication of the working group*: it is important to identify subjects to be involved and the person to be designated to manage the process (*team leader*);

2) *identification of the cases* to be analyzed according to level of risk;
3) *collection, structuring and evaluation of information:* it is a question of identifying information sources useful for understanding the causes of the event (Incident Reporting cards, clinical records, protocols, registers, interviews), organizing them chronologically and assessing their severity or less;
4) *identification of problems and causes* through tools, such as meetings, diagrams and matrices;
5) *identification of solutions and corrective and improvement activities;*
6) *final elaboration of a document* summarizing all the actions undertaken, tools used and strategic solutions adopted.

While this technique allows to actively involve professionals and share their goals, on the other hand, it can be a long and arduous process, due to the need to find, process and compare all the information required to understand the event, discerning the causes attributable to human error from those related to violations of processes and procedures.

Ishikawa diagram (or fish bone or cause-effect) is the tool that is most often used to analyze interactions between contributing factors and root causes (fig. 5.4). The main spine represents the event adverse, while the other thorns reproduce causes and contributing factors.

Fig. 5.4 Diagram of Ishikawa

Contributing factors

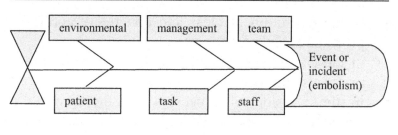

Source: adaptation by Cuzzupoli, Soccetti, Catalani, De Palma, Rischio clinico nelle fratture prossimali di femore, G.I.O.T. 2005; 31: 90-5[9]

Taking again the example described in Figure 4.8, p. 91 (case of embolism during surgery), it is possible to identify the causes attributable to some of the most relevant contributing factors, attributable to the aforementioned case:

- *Patient-related factors*: incomplete data in the patient's condition folder.
- *Factors linked to management*: deficit of data in medical record, due to lack of adequate protocols.
- *Team factors and tasks*: failed supervision of exams and graphics in the folder, for poor verbal communication between doctors and paramedics.

The good outcome of the proceeding derives, first of all, from the desire to participate and actively collaborate in all phases (starting from the leadership); secondly, by the ability to identify strategies and additional measures to optimize expected results.

This means directing improvement actions:

- in the management and structure of health records, especially medical records, to ensure completeness and reliability of the data;
- in the definition of clear and concretely applicable procedures and guidelines;
- in the correct use of equipment, through the use of protocols and recommendations;
- in the revision of processes for the training of surgical checklists, in the different surgical operative units, to reduce or eliminate incidence of errors and omissions[10] (for example regarding the correct identification of the patient and surgical site).

5.2.2 FMEA (*Failure Mode and Effect Analysis*) and FMECA (*Failure Mode, Effects and Criticality Analysis*)

FMEA and FMECA, unlike the RCA, are forecasting methods (respectively qualitative and quantitative), used to identify vulnerabilities[11], critical issues inherent in the system and the possible areas of error[12], in order to prevent adverse events and consequent damages. They are used for the systematic analysis of a process or activity, to define:
- what might not work and where (failure mode and critical areas);
- because the error or the fault could happen;
- what could be the possible effects (failure effects);[6]
- what corrections to make to secure the process or activity.

Also in this case, the analysis should be carried out by a multidisciplinary team, led by the risk manager, because of the heterogeneity of activities (fig. 5.5).

Fig. 5.5 FMEA/FMECA Process

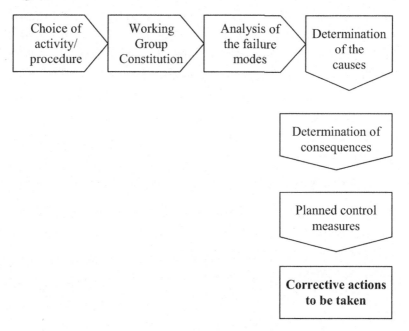

Source: adaptation by ARS Emilia Romagna, Dossier 75/2002

FMEA and FMECA use assessment techniques to estimate qualitative and quantitative risk and severity of risk (pages 92-94). The three factors taken into consideration are:
1) probability or frequency of occurrence of the error (P);
2) severity of the effects/consequences of the error (S);
3) the error detection or the possibility that it can be identified by the control measures present in the system (D)[11].

Depending on the process examined, the group decides to attribute to each element a value (for example from 1 to 10), in order to calculate Risk Priority Index:

RPI: P x S x D; min 1, max 1000. This is an essential phase, since it allows to immediately identify the area of the system most at risk (error mode with a higher RPI) and to take decisions to minimize the level of risk through control, reduction or elimination.

The following example concerns the application of this methodology in the analysis and monitoring of errors, that are more commonly found in the treatment processes for "Anesthesiological Activity" (tab. 5.4).

Tab 5.4 Example of FMEA / FMECA application in Anesthesia

PHASE OF THE PROCESS	METHODS AND CAUSES OF ERROR	CORRECTIVE ACTIONS
RECOGNITION OF EQUIPMENT	Unavailability of: - respirator - defibrillator - monitor - aspirators	- Daily Cheek before operating sessions; - Check power and connection
PHARMACIES AND PRESIDES RECOGNITION	Non-availability of drugs and devices for anesthesia and intensive care room	- Daily check of availability - Preparation of the current before each procedure
PATIENT RECOGNITION	- Patient exchange; - Documentation exchange; - Illegible writing	- Electronic identification bracelet; - Double check; - Clarity in writing
TAKING OVER PATIENT	- Failure to observe pre-operative fasting - Unavailability informed consent	- Patient questioning; - Verification of presence
POSITIONING ON THE OPERATING TABLE	Mal placement	Check position that does not cause neurovascular damage

INDUCTION AND MAINTENANCE OF ANESTHESIA	- Failure to recognize cardio respiratory problems; - Anaphylactic drug shock	- Observation of the patient; -Constant monitoring of unconsciousness and vital parameters - Appropriate tests against allergy; - Electronic bracelet reading with alarm signal
AWAKENING	Falling from the operating bed	- Check the bed attachment; - Close supervision by the staff even of the awake patient

Source: adaptation by Ministry of Health, Risk Management in Healthcare. The problem of errors, 2004

One study found[13] that (with the use of this technique) the increase in patient safety is directly proportional to the reduction in number of adverse events. In fact, the advantages attributable to it are the following (*Strengths*):

- it is used to identify and evaluate both errors of individuals and work team that the latent ones, linked to the decisions taken by management;
- it can be applied to individual activities, as in the example above or to an entire process;
- it can help reduce the length of stay;
- it can contribute to reducing the number of complaints;
- it improves the image and reputation of the organization.

Possible limitations of this technique (*Weaknesses*) are due to the following factors:

- inability to deal with defects and shortcomings found in a related manner, as if they were single units (human error, system error, etc.);
- the need to have a considerable amount of information, especially when the object of analysis is a whole process;
- need to involve heterogeneous and competent professionals, ensuring collaboration and consensus of all.

5.3 Risk treatment tools

5.3.1 The use of innovative computerized technologies to improve security and safety

In the healthcare sector, the use of advanced technologies is perhaps one of the most debated and investigated aspects regarding safety, especially if we consider the aim pursued: improvement of the system reliability and reduction of clinical and organizational risk.

In fact, implementation of new technologies can:
- favor the increase of quality and processes and activities optimization;
- improve working conditions by reducing the occurrence of errors;
- improve communication between subjects and the various organizational units, memory capacity, decision-making capacity;
- carry out routine operations in a reliable way;
- identify in advance any failures and dangerous situations, through alarm systems;

- facilitate the registration and mapping of all errors[14].

For this reason, more and more often we talk about Health Technology, understood as: "the set of prevention and rehabilitation activities, drugs, devices, medical and surgical procedures and systems, within which health is protected and maintained"[15].

It refers not only to *hard components* (such as equipment and medical devices), but also to *soft components*, related to welfare, management and technical-administrative aspects (policies and procedures, activities, communication, training)[16].

There are various technological, information and robotics solutions, integrated in healthcare systems, for accident prevention, especially in the following areas (clinical and management ones)[17]:

- drug management process, considered the major cause of errors in the hospital;
- identification of the patient and surgical sites;
- certification of the sterilization process of surgical instruments;
- management of test tubes for analysis and transfusion laboratories;
- electronic storage of clinical-administrative data, such as computerized records.

Initially, the automation and introduction of new technologies can increase the complexity of the system, producing new types of errors, especially if the systems are poorly designed and managed.

But if we consider technology as innovation and support, it can certainly contribute to making errors visible and interceptable, as well as minimizing their effects.

In particular, with regard to medication errors (Figure 5.6), strategies to reduce them are both first and second level.

Fig. 5.6 Drug Mistakes

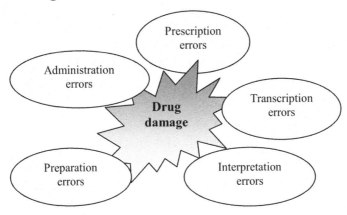

The first-level strategies are actions aimed at changing the management process as:

- double checks;
- check list;
- advice from pharmacists.

The second level ones are designed to fully computerize the process through[17]:

- computerized systems for prescription of therapy;
- decentralized computerized wardrobes;
- controlled administration by bar code;
- management systems of unit dose drug.

5.3.2 Case study: "San Raffaele Hospital, Milan"

The San Raffaele Scientific Institute of Milan has implemented a model (*Intelligent Hospital System*), which shows how the intelligent application of technologically advanced systems and optimized management of data transmission can contribute to

126

reducing the margin of error. It is a technology that includes a set of tools, such as radiofrequency identification systems, which have replaced bar code systems and smart cart.

Radiofrequency Identification System (RFID) is a wireless communication technology that uses radio waves for the automatic acquisition of information, in order to identify and monitor objects and people. This technology uses signals in the radiofrequency (RF) spectrum, to communicate data in a unidirectional and bidirectional manner between the receiving and transmitting devices[18].

The experimentation was carried out in the immune-haematology and transfusion medicine department, with the aim of significantly reducing risk of error in transfusion process, through the cross-authentication between patient's data and blood bags coding. After medical assessment, the patient is provided with a device called *transponder*, inserted in a bracelet, where his personal data and photography are recorded.

After blood collection, an electronic label is applied to the blood bag on which all patient data are transferred (from the bracelet and stored), to allow identification of collected sample. At the time of transfusion, through programmed handhelds, the congruence between data contained in the bracelet and those present in electronic label is verified.

In case of inconsistency between the data, handheld emits an alarm signal to alert operator to stop the action. Otherwise, transfusion can be performed and the Transfusional Center receives confirmation of the operation of that specific unit of blood, having an immediate control on what happens in the departments and on the signaling of any transfusion reactions[19].

On the other hand, the smart cart is equipped with a software for managing the entire drug management process and robotic drawers for the automatic delivery of medicines.

It allows an automatic identification of the patient (always through electronic bracelet), every time the prescription and delivery of drugs are performed. The reading of bracelet involves automatic opening of the drawer, where the drugs are contained for that patient, in that dose, at the right time for the administration, giving rise to alarm signals when trying to administer a drug to which the patient is allergic [20].

To ensure the effectiveness of results achieved by applying any innovative technology, it is necessary to have:

- an organizational configuration suitable to support a highly complex process;
- a network of applications and IT systems, highly integrated, ensuring a constant flow of shared information and the interaction between the different clinical departments and services;
- competence and knowledge on the correct use of new technology.

References

1. AGENZIA SANITARIA REGIONALE, Emilia Romagna, (2003), *Il sistema di Incident Reporting nelle Organizzazioni Sanitarie*, Dossier 86.

2. WORLD HEALTH ORGANIZATION, (2005), *Who draft guidelines for adverse event reporting and learning systems*.

3. www.jcaho.org

4. AGENZIA SANITARIA REGIONALE, Emilia Romagna, (2014), *Chi ascolta, cambia! Segnalazioni dei cittadini e qualità percepita nelle Aziende sanitarie*, Dossier n. 245.

5. TRIBUNALE PER I DIRITTI DEL MALATO, (2005/2006), Audit Civico, *La Valutazione delle Aziende Sanitarie realizzate dai Cittadini*.

6. MINISTERO DELLA SALUTE, Dipartimento della Qualità, (2007), *Sicurezza dei pazienti e gestione del rischio clinico: Manuale per la formazione degli operatori sanitari*.

7. ASR EMILIA ROMAGNA, (2006), *La RCA per l'analisi del rischio nelle strutture sanitarie*, Dossier 130.

8. CONFORTINI M.C.- PATRINI E., (2006), *Manuale di Risk Management in sanità processi e strumenti di implementazione*, Il Sole 24 Ore.

9. CUZZUPOLI P., SOCCETTI A., CATALANI A., DE PALMA L., (2005), *Rischio clinico nelle fratture prossimali di femore*, G.I.O.T; 31: 90-5.

10. AZIENDA OSPEDALIERA SAN FILIPPO NERI, Regione Lazio, (2007), *Piano Aziendale Unità Gestione Rischio*.

11. AGENZIA SANITARIA REGIONALE, Emilia Romagna, (2002), *FMEA - FMECA Analisi dei modi*

di errore/guasto e dei loro effetti nelle organizzazioni sanitarie, Dossier 75.

12. MINISTERO DELLA SALUTE, (2004), *Risk Management in Sanità. Il problema degli errori.*

13. LATINO ROBERT J., (2004), *Optimizing FMEA and RC in healthcare, ASHRM JOURNAL 2004*, www.proactforhealthcare.com

14. POINT OF CARE BULLETTIN, (2005), *La sicurezza dei pazienti e l'utilizzo delle nuove tecnologie. Una relazione pericolosa?* Ott. 2005.

15. POINT OF CARE BULLETTIN, (2006), *Valutazione delle tecnologie sanitarie e sicurezza dei pazienti nei sistemi di governance integrata dell'APSS di Trento*, Gennaio, n. 1.

16. POINT OF CARE BULLETTIN, (2006), *Valutazione delle tecnologie sanitarie e sicurezza dei pazienti nei sistemi di governance integrata dell'APSS di Trento*, Set., n. 2/3.

17. AGENZIA SANITARIA REGIONALE, Emilia Romagna, (2006), *Tecnologie Informatizzate per la sicurezza nell'uso dei farmaci*, Dossier n. 120.

18. AGENZIA SANITARIA REGIONALE, Emilia Romagna, (2006), *Sistemi di identificazione automatica*, Dossier n. 135.

19. ISTITUTO SCIENTIFICO UNIVERSITARIO S. RAFFAELE, MILANO, Cisco System,(2006), *L'errore in Medicina si cura con l'innovazione.*

20. OSPEDALE SAN RAFFAELE, (2003), *Il progetto Drive.*

CHAPTER 6

RISK MANAGEMENT IN INTERNATIONAL AND NATIONAL CONTEXT

Summary: 6.1 The US context from the '70s to today - 6.2 The situation in Italy. *6.2.1 National initiatives about Risk Management. 6.2.2 New rules on Risk Management and responsibility of Health professionals (Law March 8, 2017, No 24) 6.2.3 A survey on health care organizations. 6.2.3.1 Risk Management in the Italian healthcare context 6.2.3.2 Areas, tools and techniques of Risk Management* - References

6.1 The US context from the '70s to today

In the US, the problem of malpractice dates back to the early '70s, following a rapid increase in complaints against doctors and hospitals, for damages caused by medical treatment.

Risk Management System was introduced to try to contain both the negative effects (resulting from incorrect treatment) and the costs of processes and reimbursements.

Initially it concerned the methods of containing financial risk; only later it was also adopted in terms of patient and organization safety.

After a first phase in which only cases of negligence

were analyzed, a study was carried out, requested by the Nixon administration, from which concomitant causes of the error emerged:

- risks related to new technologies;
- a progressive deterioration of doctor-patient relationships;
- an increasing number of professionals involved in the single episode of care[1].

While in the '70s only a few structures had a Risk Management function, in the '80s the percentage rose to 50%. Currently, most hospitals use risk management activities not only for legal and economic reasons, but also because each damage causes an increase in health costs.

In 1980 the *American Society for Healthcare Risk Management* was born, with the aim of providing assistance to the structures in which this function was established. Subsequently, several other organizations are set up to promote security actions:

- *Agency for Healthcare Research and Quality* (AHRQ): it allocates funds for research and provides training, reports, indicators and practical guides;
- *Institute for healthcare improvement* (IHI): it promotes tangible initiatives, such as the recent "100,000 lives" campaign which, according to the literature (Ovreitveit, 2005), has prevented an average death of 115 people per year in American hospitals;
- *National Center for Patient Safety of the National Veterans Organization* which, in addition to providing resources, issues guidelines and training;
- *Joint commission* for accreditation of healthcare organizations that has developed international safety standards and reports;

- *Leapfrog group*, formed by the largest US health service entrepreneurs/buyers, with the function of measuring quality of care and efficiency with which hospitals use resources in the most at-risk clinical areas. Each hospital is assigned a score based on the results obtained in the different areas and activities. If they prove to maintain or improve their level of excellence, can achieve economic and incentive awards (for example, for the prevention and management of chronic diseases)[2].
- *Institute of Medicine* (IOM), which provides independent scientific advice to the government; it publishes reports that strongly influence the actions and decisions of the health care system, in terms of safety.

The Health Security Action Plan was decided and approved by US Government, following publication of the shock report *"To err is human"* in which, since 1999, it was reported:
- the death of 45,000 - 98,000 Americans every year, due to medical errors that could be foreseen and avoided;
- the damage caused to about one million Americans every year;
- costs for errors and damages, of approximately 29 billion dollars.

In 2000 the Agency for Research and Quality of care (in collaboration with several organizations involved in the healthcare security) published the Report *"Federal action to reduce medical errors and their impact"*[3]. It contains a series of actions, directed to all healthcare facilities, to identify and study the causes of error and implement preventive and corrective actions.

According to the *"Learning for Errors"* report, the principle on which all intervention actions should be planned is *"learning from mistakes"*. An effective reporting system was therefore implemented, first applied as a pilot project in 500 hospitals and clinics and later extended to most of healthcare organizations.

The program included:

- an active involvement of leadership and of all health workers;
- the confidentiality of the report, to be used to prevent and not to punish;
- a continuous feedback between federal agencies and hospitals, in order to create a database of integrated information on documented errors, to be interpreted through regular meetings;
- use of the most appropriate technology to support medical practice;
- the use of checklists and standardized procedures, for example in management of drug process or in the operating room (hand washing, cap, gown, mask and full barrier cloths).

In this context, the federal healthcare system continues to support healthcare organizations in the continuous improvement of quality, including through provision and implementation of training programs and critical learning.

The AHRQ has launched a newspaper on the web, where doctors can submit errors, having as guarantee the respect of anonymity, useful for educating patients and operators. This has shown that case studies are very effective for raising general awareness about the safety issue and for training physicians on specific topics.

Several American hospitals (including Vanderbilt Hospital) have implemented 360-degree Risk Management systems.

They provide for dissemination of guides and manuals on the main procedures to follow for event reporting, the correct information to patients and operators, the release to patients of a copy of the medical records, the management of communication between health personnel and family members (Source: *https://ww2.mc.vanderbilt.edu*).

Regarding the current situation, it is interesting the annual report, published by the Health Grades on Quality, in American Hospitals. It analyzes the number of accidents and results achieved in the quality of care in 4.500 healthcare organizations.

In 2014, the best hospitals were identified in achieving clinical excellence, improving patient safety and achieving better performance compared to other hospitals, both in terms of the number of accidents and the number of deaths[4].

This report shows that the overall change in recent years has been significant and that changes in quality of care increase considerably, also thanks to the development and dissemination of public guides and reports. However, variations in clinical outcomes continue to exist, even within the same city.

This implies that it should not be taken for granted that the nearest hospital represents the best structure, if it does not have the most suitable procedures for that type of operation.

Furthermore, the use of minimally invasive surgical techniques can significantly contribute to reduce mortality and patient's stay in the structure and simultaneously to reduce overall costs of hospital care and direct costs.

The analysis shows that 234,252 lives could potentially be saved and 157,418 complications could potentially be avoided. The ultimate goal is to reduce errors by 50%, urging the parties concerned to report the error as soon as possible and to talk openly about their mistakes, at least between doctors (as happens in the

"*Commission deaths*", convened once a week, behind closed doors, to study errors and not repeat them again).

Therefore every subject, within the structure, is directly responsible for their role and for carrying out their activities, to improve results and reduce costs. Communication is the key element to ensure value and quality of health care.

6.2 The situation in Italy

6.2.1 National initiatives about Risk Management

In Italy, for many years, Risk Management has been the subject of many initiatives by the Italian Regions, interested in developing a set of tools and activities to support safety in healthcare organizations.

In this context, the Ministry of Health established in 2003 the Technical Commission on Clinical Risk, with the specific role of drawing up a document that formulated general guidelines and recommendations on risk management: "*Risk Management in Healthcare. The problem of errors*".

Also in 2003, the Ministry carried out a national survey on "*initiatives for patient safety*", referring to 2002, by administering a questionnaire, aimed at all healthcare structures, to verify the policies promoted within risk management[5].

Between 2008 and 2014, several recommendations were developed and published, with the specific aim of raising awareness, guiding decision-making choices of healthcare organizations and providing effective tools to reduce risks.

The most relevant are the following ones (tab. 6.1):

Tab. 6.1 Recommendations 2005-2014

N.	Title	Date
17	Reconciliation of drug therapy	Dec. 2014
16	Recommendation to prevent death or permanent disability in healthy newborn weighing> 2500 grams, unrelated to congenital disease	Apr. 2014
15	Death or serious damage resulting from an incorrect assignment of the triage code in the Operations Center 118 and/or in the Emergency Room	Feb. 2013
14	Prevention of errors in therapy with antineoplastic drugs	Nov. 2012
13	Prevention and management of patient fall in health facilities	Nov. 2011
12	Prevention of errors in therapy with "Look-alike/sound-alike" drugs	Aug. 2010
11	Death or serious damage resulting from a malfunction of the transport system (intra-hospital, extra hospital). N.B. The Recommendation has been brought to the attention of the Coordination of Regions and Autonomous Provinces for Patients Safety, for which it could undergo modifications	Jan. 2010
10	Prevention of bisphosphonate jaw osteonecrosis	Sep. 2009
9	Prevention of adverse events resulting from the failure of medical devices/electro-medical devices	Apr. 2009
8	Preventing acts of violence against health workers	Nov. 2007
7	Prevention of death, coma or severe harm resulting from errors in drug therapy	Mar. 2008
6	Prevention of maternal death related to labor and / or delivery	Mar. 2008
5	Prevention of the transfusion reaction from incompatibility of the AB0 group	Mar. 2008

4	Prevention of suicide of a patient in a hospital	Mar.2008
3	Correct identification of patients, surgical site and procedure	Mar. 2008
2	Preventing the retention of gauze, instruments or other material within the surgical site	Mar. 2008
1	Correct use of concentrated solutions of Potassium Chloride -KCL- and other concentrated solutions containing Potassium	Mar. 2008

Source: Ministry of Health, 2014

On 20 February 2006 a *Patient Safety Working Group* was set up by decree, with the task to:[6]

- develop a system for monitoring adverse events and insurance policies;
- develop a manual on analysis of errors and strategies for training implementation, aimed at all healthcare professionals and published in May 2007 on the Ministry of Health website;
- provide techniques and tools for an active patient involvement.

In this regard in March 2007, for the first time, the *Working Table on Patient Safety* met with the representatives of the *Citizens Forum*[7]. It is a body set up in 2001 at the Department for Health and brings together organizations representing the interests of NHS users, with the function to:

- verify the strategies and activities carried out by the Local Health Authorities in terms of safety, through the mandatory presentation of annual reports;
- identify effective practices for security to be spread annually;
- identify suitable training paths;

- interact and learn about initiatives undertaken by regional commissions.

On January 10th of the same year, the Reference National System for Patient Safety was set up, activated experimentally for a period of two years, at the Ministry of Health. It is a tool through which all healthcare professionals can obtain information regarding safety and avoidable events of particular relevance. It should also facilitate monitoring and exchange of information and reports, by sharing knowledge acquired within the healthcare system.

In May, in collaboration with the National Federation of the Order of Physicians, Surgeons and Dentists and the National Federation of Nursing Colleges, the first distance course for healthcare workers was organized on *Safety of Care and Clinical Risk Government*.

In 2011 the Guidelines for *"managing and communicating adverse events in healthcare"* were issued, following the activation of *"Monitoring protocol for sentinel events"*, aimed at identifying ways of monitoring and managing events in Italy in collaboration with the Regions.

In 2012 the Ministry of Health established the Information System for Monitoring of Errors in Health Care (SIMES), with "the aim of gathering information about sentinel events and complaints claims throughout the country, by allowing the assessment of risks and a full monitoring of adverse events" (Ministry of Health website)[8].

The SIMES consists of two components (sentinel event management and claims management) and it is organized on three levels of intervention that work synergistically:

1) monitoring, through which all information regarding sentinel events and claims for risk assessment is acquired;
2) recommendations elaborated on the basis of information collected through monitoring, aimed at identifying the actions needed to improve quality of care;
3) staff training, useful for acquiring a greater awareness and knowledge for the improvement of patient safety methods and tools.

All the organizational structures of the NHS are responsible for the process of collecting data and information that flows into the SIMES Information System. "Following the activation of the SIMES, starting from 1° January 2009, all the Regions use the SIMES application providing for the validation of events entered by the respective organizations.

Instead, the National Observatory for the Monitoring of Sentinel Events intervenes for final validation, which allows the inclusion of data validated in the final reports" (Ministry of Health website).

Information acquired through the SIMES is used to elaborate *Sentinel Monitoring Reporting Reports* (tab. 3.14, p. 68), useful for implementing actions and changes aimed at reducing the probability of occurrence of such events.

6.2.2 New rules on Risk Management and responsibility of health professionals (Law March 8, 2017, No. 24)[9]

With the introduction of the Gelli law (Law March 8, 2017, No. 24), the adoption of a Risk Management model, in all public and private healthcare structures, has been made obligatory, with the aim of monitoring, preventing and managing punctually all hypothetical risk scenarios.

In particular, article 1 states that "all personnel are required to contribute to the risk prevention activities, implemented by public and private healthcare facilities, including self-employed professionals who work under the agreement with the National Health Service".

The other highlights of the law are described below.

- **Ombudsman.** In particular, the figure of the Ombudsman was introduced. It can be assigned the role of ensuring the right to health, at the discretion of the regions and autonomous provinces. Any recipient of health services can resort to it, in order to report malfunctions of the healthcare system. When it finds that the report is well founded, it acts to protect the right violated, in accordance with the guidelines established by regional legislation (art. 2).

- **Center for health risk management and patient safety.** It is established in each Region with the task of: 1) collecting data and information on risks, adverse events and disputes from all public and private structures and 2) transmitting them annually to the National Observatory of Good Practices on Health Safety (Article 2) .

- **National observatory of good practices on health care safety.** It operates within the National Agency for Regional Health Services (AGENAS) with the aim of acquiring the above data, but also to identify preventive measures, management and monitoring of good practices for the safety of care (art. 3), (http://buonepratiche.agenas.it/).

- **Data transparency.** All services provided must be subject to the requirement of transparency and each structure must publish on their websites the data relating to "all the compensation paid over the last

141

five years, verified in the context of the monitoring, prevention and health risk management" (art. 4).

- The law redefines civil and penal liability by extending the concept beyond medical personnel and due to all healthcare professionals (articles 6-7).

In particular, regarding the penal liability, the new art. 590 sexies provides that "if the event has occurred due to inexperience, punishment is excluded when the recommendations of the guidelines (as defined and published in accordance with law) are respected or, failing that, the good clinical and welfare practices are respected, always that recommendations, provided by the aforementioned guidelines, are appropriate to the specificities of the concrete case".

6.2.3 A survey on healthcare organizations

6.2.3.1 Risk Management in the Italian healthcare context

During 2011 and 2014, a nationwide survey was carried out, using a questionnaire, to assess the implementation of innovative management models in healthcare organizations.

Here we will be presented the most significant results considered for analysis.

All the respondents stated that they use one or more management methods and the analysis shows that the most widespread one is represented by *Risk Management*, applied partially or globally in 100% of cases, followed by *Total Quality Management* (33 % of total structures), *Balanced Scorecard* (28%) and *Business Process Reengineering* (5%) (fig. 6.1)[10].

Fig. 6.1 The management methods used

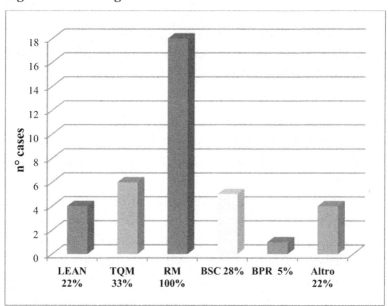

Source: Raimondo C., (2014), p. 193

All companies have given a significant importance to prevention and risk management activities in healthcare, with a positive correlation between the orientation of their decisions, choices and actions towards continuous improvement of company processes, the organizational quality and healthcare one and cultural growth of the whole organization, starting from leadership.

The latter is believed to be the most important element for the development of an effective internal and external relational network, a necessary condition for encouraging the implementation of innovative management models.

In all the companies analyzed, a partial or global Risk Management program has been implemented, while only some organizations have declared to resort to other innovative management methods and tools aimed at reducing waste (Lean Management Model) and to identify:

- paths of improvement throughout the organization;
- systems to control organizational aspects and relationships with the user (*Total Quality Management* e *Balanced Scorecard*).

Risk Management was the most operational model, because it provides the most suitable tools for detection and analysis of risks, to ensure the safety of patients and operators.

During 2014, again through a questionnaire, two other companies were contacted (Brindisi and Novara hospitals). The results were included in the table and in the following graphs, along with the results related to other healthcare companies.

Tab. 6.2 *Risk Management* **in Italian healthcare organizations**

ASL ASCOLI PICENO (MARCHE)	
Areas involved	**Areas to involve**
Risk Management in all clinical departments and health services: • Implementation of a single therapeutic card; • Report sheet for incident reporting, adverse events and accidental falls, implementation of analytical tools; • FMEA and RCA identification	

ASL BRINDISI (PUGLIA), 2014	
Areas involved	**Areas to involve**
Medical and surgical area, drug management, transfusions, hospital infections, health records, staff training	Surgical Unit or Operating block

ASL CHIETI (ABRUZZO)	
Areas involved	**Areas to involve**
The whole company	

ASL FIRENZE (TOSCANA)	
Areas involved	**Areas to involve**
Clinical Risk Management for all the Company's facilities. Risk Management Project in all departments of the 6 Hospitals	

ASL NAPOLI (CAMPANIA)	
Areas involved	**Areas to involve**
Risk Management in Operating Room, Surgery Department (5 Hospitals), District Operating Units (Health Care Operative Unit of Base), Departments of clinical pathology and Radiology, through: • Risk assessment committee; • Implementation of the Claims Assessment Committee; • Monitoring implementation of sentinel event and claims (through SIMES - Information System for Monitoring Health Errors); • Organizational well-being participation	

ASL NUORO (SARDEGNA)	
Areas involved	**Areas to involve**
The whole company	

ASL PARMA (EMILIA ROMAGNA)	
Areas involved	**Areas to involve**
Risk Management: the reporting of sentinel events, prevention of biological risk, errors analysis and management of litigation involve all the company's departments across the board. *Incident Reporting* is adopted in 4 of the 5 hospital departments. In the operating room, safety procedures are adopted in the two surgical departments. In pharmacology therapy, safety, falls prevention and informed consent to healthcare are adopted in the five hospital departments and in the mental health department. The prevention of acts of violence on operators is subject to implementation in the two first-aid units and in the mental health and pathological addictions department.	*Incident reporting*: all hospital and territorial departments. Expansion risk map: all departments, both hospital and territorial ones. Specific procedures on the safety of patients and operators in the various operating units/ departments.

ASL RAGUSA (SICILIA)	
Areas involved	**Areas to involve**
Department of Services, First Aid	

ASL RIETI (Lazio)	
Areas involved	**Areas to involve**
The whole company	

TRENTO (Trentino Alto Adige)	
Areas involved	**Areas to involve**
The whole company	

AO DESENZANO (Lombardia)	
Areas involved	**Areas to involve**
The whole company	

AO LODI (Lombardia)	
Areas involved	**Areas to involve**
The whole company	

AO PADOVA (Veneto)	
Areas involved	**Areas to involve**
All departments	

AO NOVARA (Piemonte), 2014	
Areas involved	**Areas to involve**
Medical and surgical area, obstetrics, operating room/surgery, drug management, transfusion, hospital infections	Gradual extension to all departments

AOU S.G. BATTISTA TORINO (Piemonte)	
Areas involved	**Areas to involve**
All departments	

AOU MODENA (Emilia Romagna)	
Areas involved	**Areas to involve**
The projects involve all departments of the company, but with methods and degree of variable involvement. Management is always involved	

OSPEDALE GARBAGNATE RHO (Lombardia)	
Areas involved	**Areas to involve**
Risk Management active for 3 years: General and Specialized Medicine, General and Specialist Surgery with the introduction of Week Surgery, Department of Emergency and Acceptance (DEA), Laboratory of analysis - Radiology - Medical Directions (medical)	DEA, Maternal Infantile, Services, Psychiatry, Rehabilitation

OSPEDALE LATISANA (Friuli-Venezia Giulia)	
Areas involved	**Areas to involve**
Surgical Department - Emergency Area, Maternal-Infant Department	Medical Department

IRCCS ISTITUTO EUROPEO ONCOLOGIA (Milano)	
Areas involved	**Areas to involve**
The whole Institute	

Source: processing of questionnaires by Raimondo C., (2014)

All the companies have said to use the risk management model. However, it emerged that part of them expects to extend it in all areas and departments, where 11 of them have adopted a global and integrated risk management program, throughout the organization (fig. 6.2).

Fig. 6.2 The total/partial adoption of Risk Management model

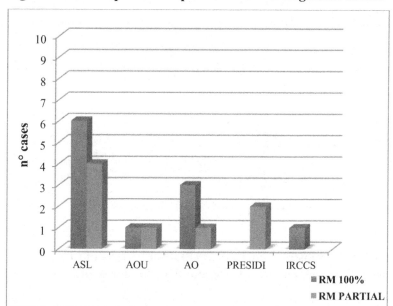

ASL: Azienda Sanitaria Locale (Local Health Company).
AOU: Azienda Ospedaliera Universitaria (University Hospital).
AO: Azienda Ospedaliera (Hospital Company).
Presidi/Ospedali: Hospital Garrison (it is a hospital not set up in a Hospital Company, as it does not meet the legal requirements. It has a very minor autonomy.
IRCCS: Istituto di Ricovero e Cura a Carattere Scientifico (Institute of Hospitalization and Care with a Scientific Character).

With regard to the timing for implementing Risk Management projects, 5 healthcare companies have stated different implementation times, characterized by a significant variability (fig. 6.3).

This variability is likely to be correlated with barriers eventually found in the implementation phase, mainly due to cultural factors (resistance to change), lack of a clear and shared strategy and lack of resources and limited budget (fig. 6.4).

149

Fig. 6.3 The timing of implementation of Risk Management projects

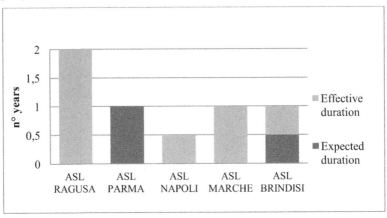

Fig. 6.4 (a) Obstacles to implementation by type of projects (Risk Management and Total Quality Management)

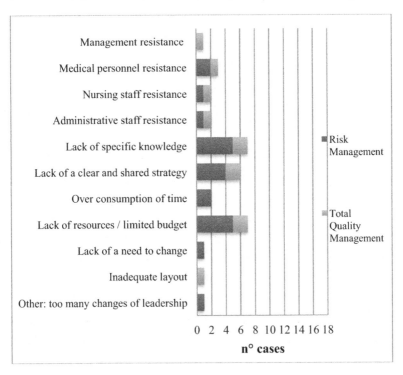

Fig. 6.4 (b) Obstacles to implementation by type of projects (Balanced Scorecard and Lean Thinking)

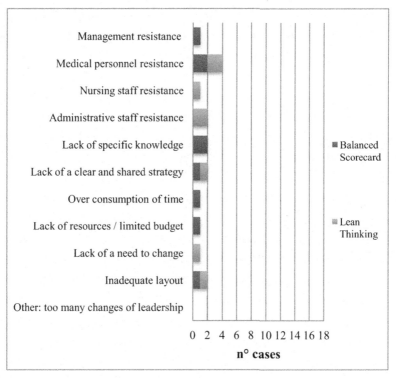

Source: processing of questionnaires by Raimondo C., (2014)

Subsequently, the referees were asked to indicate the strategies adopted, to make the personnel to a real involvement and participation in the project management activities (fig. 6.5).

Fig. 6.5 Staff engagement strategies

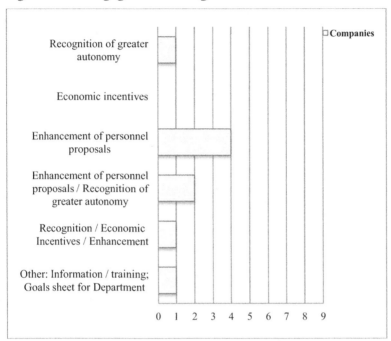

Most of the structures use strategies to *"enhance staff proposals"*. It takes on a significant value when it is recognized:

- an adequate margin of decisional and operational autonomy in the exercise of activity;
- a greater responsibility for the objectives to be achieved;
- an improvement of motivational and relational aspect, considered a strategic quality factor and an essential condition for ensuring patient/user satisfaction.

If we analyze the data related to the *"economic incentives"* dimension, we note that it has not been assigned a strategic value. This shows that apparently economic aspects impact less on staff behavior, compared to those related to motivation, which is instead associated with the enhancement of professionalism and active involvement in company management.

6.2.3.2 Areas, tools and techniques of Risk Management

With reference to the companies contacted in 2014 (which we will indicate with X and Y to protect their identity, for the purposes of recording and presenting the results), additional data have emerged regarding:
1) areas deemed most at risk;
2) areas where risk management projects were implemented;
3) adoption of tools for reporting errors;
4) risk management techniques.

Regarding the first point, only one company has provided an answer; the other structure, for reasons of privacy, declined to rule.

Tab. 6.3 Areas deemed to be at risk for the Company X

Medical area
Surgical area
Obstetrics
Orthopedics
Emergency/Operating room
Medication management
Hospital infections

The data are basically in line with analysis results of the areas that generate more requests for damages, in both civil and penal law (p. 56 and following).

As can be seen from Tables 6.3 and 6.4, there is a correlation between areas considered most at risk and implementation of Risk Management projects in the same areas, with the exception of *"Orthopedics"* area.

Tab. 6.4 Areas of implementation of Risk Management projects

Company X	Company Y
Medical area	Medical area
Surgical area	Surgical Area
Obstetrics	
Operating room	
Medication management	Medication management
Hospital infections	Hospital infections
Transfusions	Transfusions
	Health documentation
	Personnel training

Below, the tools and techniques most frequently adopted by companies, for analysis, reporting and risk management, have been identified.

From the analysis of the following table (6.5) it is possible to highlight how the main tools used (to promptly report errors) are *Incident Reporting, Sentinel Events protocol, clinical audits* and the establishment of *databases for claims and disputes.*

Tab. 6.5 Adoption of tools for reporting errors

Company X	Company Y
Incident reporting	Incident reporting
Sentinel Events	Sentinel Events
Clinical Audit	
Creation of a database for complaints and disputes	Creation of a database for complaints and disputes

Finally, table 6.6 shows that only one company (X) uses all risk management techniques, at the same time.

Tab. 6.6 Risk Management Techniques

Company X	Company Y
RCA - Root Cause Analysis	
FMEA-FMECA	FMEA-FMECA
Review and analysis of medical records	
Analysis of Hospital Discharge Cards	

From this we can deduce the presence of an integrated risk management system, aimed at the optimization of company standards and of qualitative level, through the testing of activities of causes analysis, that are subtended to the root of errors and risks emerging in the business processes.

References

1. MARCON G., (2000), *Errori e danni nelle cure mediche: USA e Regno Unito lanciano l'allarme*, Risk Management, Rischio Sanità.

2. OVRETVEIT in SIQUAS, (2006) - *Raccomandazioni sulla gestione del rischio clinico.*

3. QuIC, Report of the Quality Interagency Coordination Task, (2000), *Doing What Counts for Patient Safety: Federal Action to reduce Medical Errors and their impact*, February.

4. HEALTHGRADES REPORT, (2014), *American Hospital Quality Outcomes.*

5. MINISTERO DELLA SALUTE, (2002), *Rilevazione nazionale sulle iniziative per la sicurezza del paziente nelle strutture nel SSN.*

6. CIAMPALINI S., (2006), *Gestione del Rischio clinico e sicurezza dei pazienti: il programma del Ministero della Salute in collaborazione con le Regioni e le Aziende Sanitarie*, XXVII Congresso Nazionale SIFO (La prevenzione e la cura del paziente nelle politiche sanitarie regionali), Genova 27-30 Settembre.

7. TARTAGLIA R., MENCHINI M., (2007), *Errori, pazienti controllori*, Sanità, il Sole 24 Ore, Toscana, 24-30 Aprile.

8. MINISTRY OF HEALTH WEBSITE, System for Monitoring Errors in Health Care (Sistema Informativo per il Monitoraggio degli Errori in Sanità - SIMES).

9. Law March 8, 2017, No. 24.

10. RAIMONDO C., (2014), *Lean Innovation in Healthcare, Principles, Theories and Case Studies*, CreateSpace Independent Publishing Platform.

CONCLUSION

Most of the healthcare organizations deal with the issue of health risk and errors, through a study and an in-depth analysis of its multidimensional aspect, starting initiatives aimed at deepening the context in which it is inserted.

The main problem is to evaluate if:

a. the information acquired enables to build a comprehensive picture of the situation;

b. it is possible to compare the data, in order to have a consistent view of the phenomenon;

c. the structures and individuals are able to effectively use the tools to quickly identify the risks involved in each operation and cope with the resulting errors.

In fact, the means to act exist; however, the greatest concern is to build a system of interaction, in order to identify the best solutions, carefully defining the priorities for action to limit the risk.

It has been suggested by many parties to adopt an holistic, integrated and homogeneous approach to the problem; but in this context it is necessary to know individual regions and healthcare organizations, whose policies and positions, (relative to risk management), are often different from each other.

The simple creation of commissions, working groups and bodies of inquiry on healthcare service (to deal with the "*health risk*" issue) is insufficient. Indeed, concrete solutions to a heterogeneous and complex phenomenon must have been identified.

Currently the only really workable tool is risk mapping, applied to the healthcare system. On the one hand, it allows to photograph the real situation existing and previous experience, through the acquisition of data relating to the patient, the behavior of health workers, the suitability of structures and organization; on the other hand, to make an internal and external comparison (benchmarking), at the level of a single company or of organizations at a territorial level. The general application would favor a constructive comparison and a continuous improvement of the existing situation.

It is necessary to develop preventive programs, concerning both the quality of healthcare services provided and those related to the *"patient management"* in its broadest sense: from its hospitality and stay in the structure, to the compilation of medical record, up to the collection of informed consent.

The active involvement and awareness of all actors, in the clinical and organizational risk management process, requires a precise knowledge of the phenomenon. This knowledge is an essential process to act effectively, leaving the defensive strategy increasingly pursued (*concealing errors and denying the evidence*), by developing strategies that improve perception of the user/patient, about services quality and services provided (*promptly report the error so as not to repeat it further*).

Regardless of the activity actually carried out and services offered, one of the objectives pursued by each company is to improve security. It can be achieved through:

a. the breaking down of *"safety barriers"* (such as the excess of professional rules and the progressive accumulation over time of conflicting organizational rules, which create an unreasonable increase in the complexity of the system, without any advantage);
b. the raising of *"risk barriers"* to reduce accidents, where it is not possible to completely cancel them.

Made in the USA
Las Vegas, NV
26 March 2023

69708032R00089